EFFORTLESS
PALEO

DINNER EDITION

50 Fast and Simple Dinner Recipes

MELISSA TAYLOR

TABLE OF CONTENTS

SWEET AND SAVORY CHICKEN: MAPLE MUSTARD ALMOND CHICKEN

One unique way in making your favorite Almond Chicken is to add some sweet taste to it.

MAKES 4 SERVING/ TOTAL TIME 40 MINUTE

INGREDIENTS

2 tbsp Dijon mustard

1 tbsp Pure maple syrup

1/2 tsp Cider vinegar

1/2 cup Almonds (coarsely chopped)

4 Boneless skinless chicken breast (pounded to an even thickness)

Sea salt and fresh ground pepper (to taste)

METHOD

STEP 1

Preheat oven to 375 degrees F.

Whisk the mustard, maple syrup, and vinegar in a small bowl.

STEP 2

Add a pinch of salt and pepper to the almonds.

Brush each chicken breast with the mixture and roll in the chopped almonds.

Lay on a baking sheet and bake for 20 to 25 minutes, until chicken is cooked through and browned.

NUTRITION VALUE	331 Kcal, 20g fat, 5g fiber, 22g protein, 13g carbs.

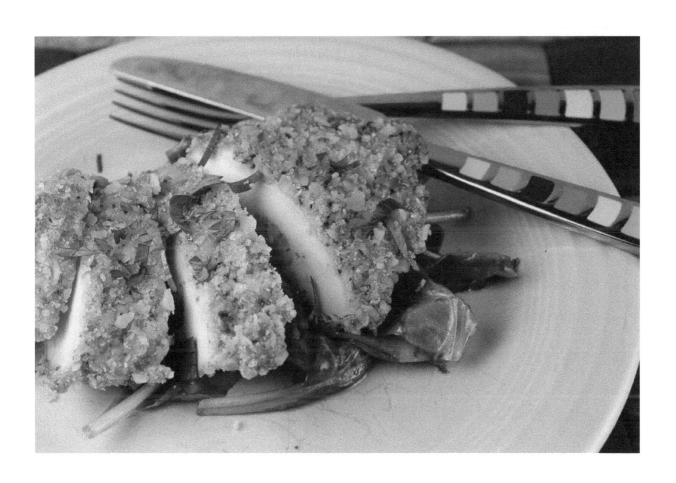

ZAB SOUP (ZUCCHINI, ARUGULA, BASIL)

The first vegetable ingredient, Zucchini, is a very versatile vegetable. It is a very low calorie vegetable – good for low calorie diet.

MAKES 1 SERVING/ TOTAL TIME 10 MINUTE

INGREDIENTS

1 Onion (medium, diced)

2 tbsp olive oil

5 Garlic cloves

3 Zucchini (medium to large)

2 cups Vegetable stock

1 pinch Salt

1 cup Fresh basil leaves (packed)

1 cup Arugula (packed)

1 Lemon (juiced)

METHOD

STEP 1

In a large pot, heat oil on high. Add diced onion and sauté until tender (3 to 4 minute) .

Chop garlic and add to pot, turn heat to medium-low for 5 minute. Slice zucchini, add to pot. Add in lemon juice and pinch of salt.

STEP 2

Bring pot contents to a simmer over high-heat, cover, turn heat down to low, and simmer 5 minutes.

After 5 minutes stir contents and cook for another 10 minutes (or until zucchini is tender) .

Pour soup into a blender or large food processor, adding the fresh basil and arugula directly into the blender (be cautious not to over fill blending device and always cover the top with a kitchen towel).

Garnish with chopped basil and hot sauce—if you like a little heat, like I do.

NUTRITION VALUE	464 Kcal, 20g fat, 20.8g fiber, 43g protein, 8g carbs.

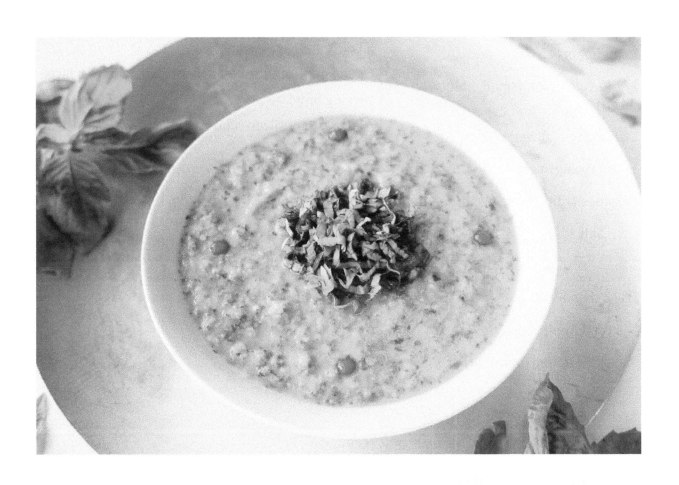

WINTER BEET SALAD

Beets are a delicious and often overlooked addition to a salad.

INGREDIENTS

1 can Beets (15 oz)

1/2 Purple onion (small , thinly sliced)

2 c Cabbage (sliced)

1 tbsp Orange zest

1 Orange (thinly sliced, skin removed)

1 tsp Salt

2 tbsp Fresh parsley (chopped)

1 1/2 tbsp EVOO

1/2 tbsp Apple cider vinegar

Drizzle of honey (optional)

METHOD

STEP 1

Open and drain the can of beets, and add to a large serving bowl.

Add in thinly sliced onion, cabbage, orange zest, and orange. Mix gently.

STEP 2

Sprinkle with salt, EVOO, parsley, vinegar, and honey. Toss.

Serve with more fresh chopped parsley as a garnish if desired.

NUTRITION VALUE	353 Kcal, 15g fat, 8g fiber, 35g protein, 15g carbs.

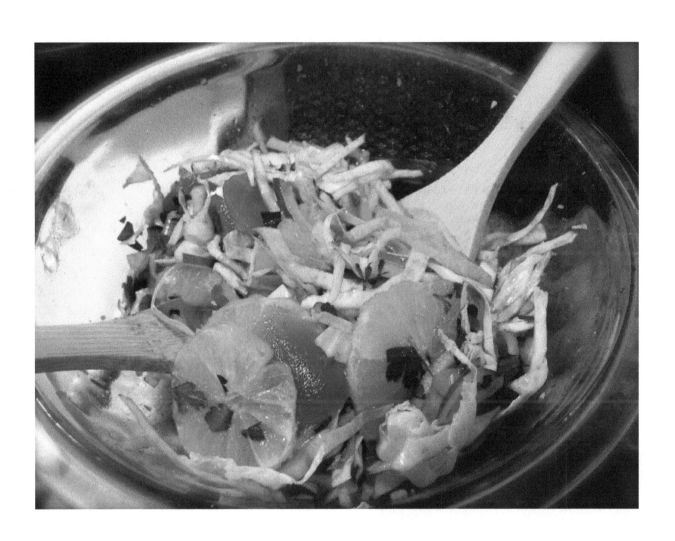

BEEF AND BROCCOLI

The flavor in this recipe is brought out with the orange juice and vinegar.

MAKES 2 SERVING/ TOTAL TIME 20 MINUTE

INGREDIENTS

1 Round steak (cut into strips)

1 cup Broccoli (cut into florets)

1 Orange

2 tbsp Apple cider vinegar

1/2 Ginger (minced)

Sea salt and black pepper (to taste)

Coconut oil

METHOD

STEP 1

Add the coconut to a medium skillet over medium-high heat. Add the round steak to the hot skillet and sauté for 3 to 4 minutes.

Add the broccoli, juice from the orange, apple cider, and ginger.

STEP 2

Season with salt and pepper.

Continue to sauté until the steak is cooked to desired temperature.

NUTRITION VALUE	358 Kcal, 20g fat, 4.5g fiber, 26.1g protein, 11.6g carbs.

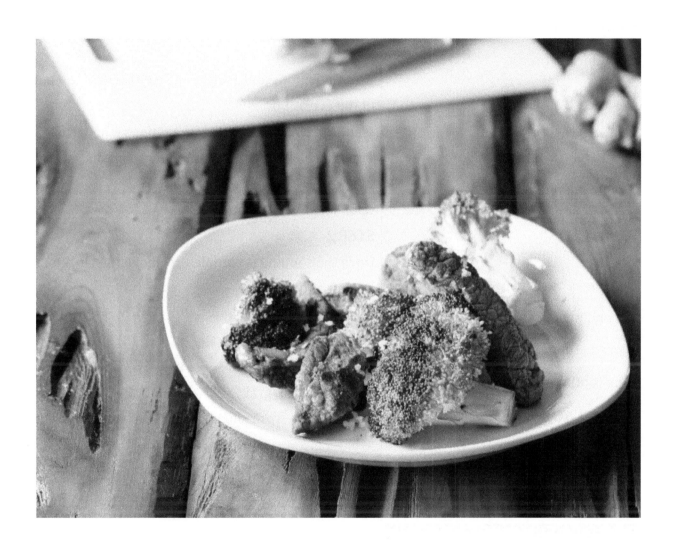

JALAPEÑO CROCK-POT PULLED CHICKEN

This Jalapeño Crock-Pot Pulled Chicken would be great on top of a salad or stuffed in a sweet potato.

MAKES 6 SERVING/ TOTAL TIME 10 MINUTE

INGREDIENTS

2 lbs Chicken breast

1 Small onion (diced)

2 Garlic cloves (minced)

16 oz Green salsa ("clean")

2 tbsp Chili powder

1 tbsp Cumin

1 sliced Jalapeno

1 c Bone broth*

Salt and pepper (to taste)

Avocado (optional)

Lime (optional)

Cilantro (optional)

METHOD

STEP 1

Dice the onions and garlic and layer them in the bottom of the Crock-Pot.

Place the chicken on top of the onions and garlic.

Top the chicken with seasonings, green salsa, and bone broth.

Cook on low for 8 hours.

STEP 2

Once the cooking is complete, remove the chicken from the pot and set aside.

Remove the liquid that is left in the Crock-Pot. That will be our salsa/gravy.

Shred the chicken and serve with avocado and the reserved salsa/gravy.

Garnish with fresh sliced jalapeño, cilantro, and lime.

NUTRITION VALUE

346 Cal, 13g fat, 3g saturated fat, 2g fiber, 47g protein, 9g carbs.

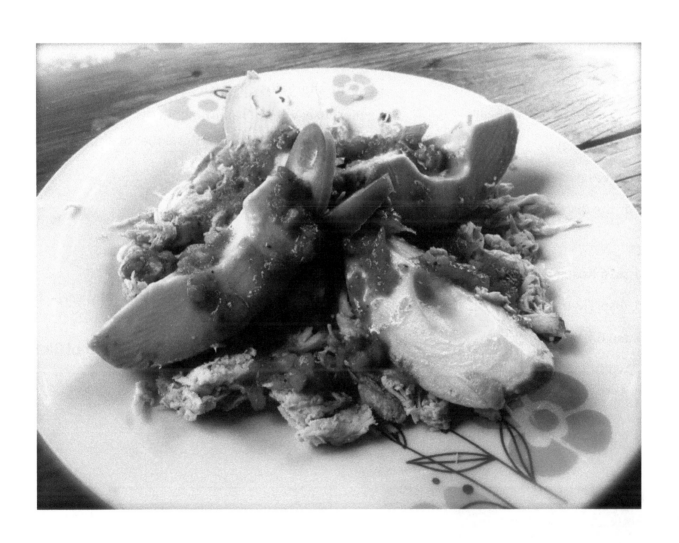

SLOW COOKER BALSAMIC SHORT RIBS

Ribs cut into short slices and pressure-cooked in a slow cooker – this is the Short Ribs Slow Cooker with Balsamic vinegar recipe.

MAKES 4 SERVING/ TOTAL TIME 10 MINUTE

INGREDIENTS

2.5 lbs Bone-in beef short ribs

1-2 tbsp Coconut oil

1 15- oz can Tomato sauce

1/2 cup Balsamic vinegar

1 tbsp Honey

6 cloves garlic (smashed)

For the dry rub

2 tbsp Salt

1 tbsp Rosemary (dried)

1 tbsp Thyme (dried)

2 tsp Garlic powder

1 tsp Onion powder

1 tsp Smoked paprika

1 tsp Freshly ground pepper

METHOD

STEP 1

In a small bowl, stir together all of the ingredients for the spice rub.

Pat the short ribs dry with a paper towel and rub generously with the spice mixture.

Melt the coconut oil in a large skillet over medium-high heat.

STEP 2

Working in batches, sear the short ribs for 2-3 minutes per side.

Place into the slow cooker.

Add the tomato sauce, balsamic, honey, and garlic to the slow cooker with the short ribs.

Cover and cook on low heat for 5-6 hours until the beef is tender.

Serve warm.

NUTRITION VALUE	646 Cal, 19g fat, 11g saturated fat, 4g fiber, 46g protein, 14g carbs.

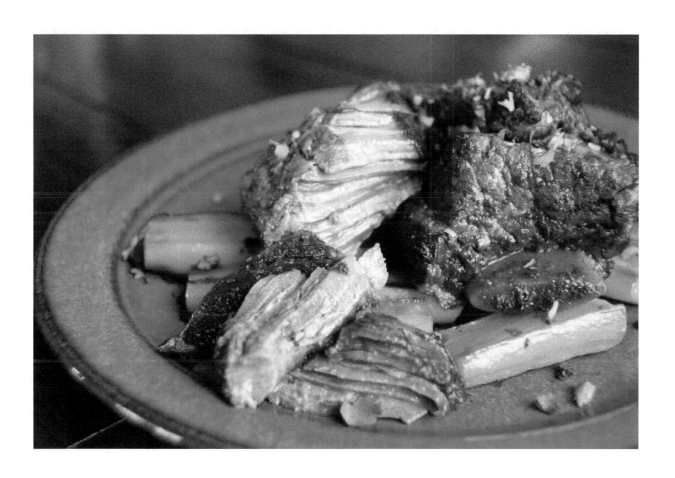

PALEO PULLED PORK & BROCCOLI

This slow cooker dish takes boring pork and turns it into an exciting dinner in just a few steps.

MAKES 4 SERVING/ TOTAL TIME 10 MINUTE

INGREDIENTS

1 lb Pork (feel free to use a cut that would be too tough to cook any other way)

1/2 c Onions (shredded)

1/2 c Cabbage (shredded)

1 tsp Garlic powder

1 tsp Onion powder

Sea salt and fresh ground pepper (to taste)

1/2 c Water

1 c Broccoli florets

Cayenne pepper (optional)

Coconut aminos (optional)

Ginger (Fresh grated - optional)

METHOD

STEP 1

Add everything but broccoli to Crock-Pot and cook on low for 8 hours or until pork falls off easily.
Once the pork is done, use 2 forks to shred the meat and mix everything together.

STEP 2

Add broccoli florets into the Crock-Pot for about 15 minutes or until they are steamed and warmed through. Garnish with cayenne pepper, coconut aminos, and fresh grated ginger.

NUTRITION VALUE

355 Cal, 19g fat, 7g saturated fat, 3g fiber, 34g protein, 10g carbs.

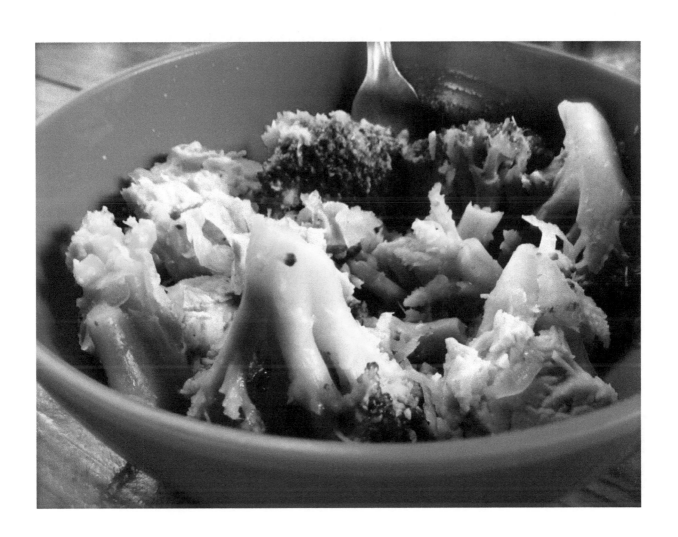

PALEO CALAMARI

Paleo calamari is here! You can have your crunch and calamari too!

INGREDIENTS

3-4 Squids (cleaned, scored and sliced into rings and tentacles)

1/4 cup Coconut flour

2 Eggs (beaten)

4 tbsp Coconut oil (for frying)

Paleo tomato sauce

METHOD

STEP 1

Add the squid to the eggs, toss to coat.

In a separate bowl, add the squid and coconut flour.

Toss to coat. Set aside while oil heats.

Add the oil to a high-sided skillet or pan over medium-high heat.

STEP 2

Add the calamari to the hot oil. Be careful, it will splatter.

Cook on each side 3 to 4 minutes, or until golden brown.

Set aside on a paper towel lined plate.

Serve with tomato sauce for dipping.

NUTRITION VALUE

327 Cal, 19g fat,
13.6g fiber, 20g protein, 14g carbs.

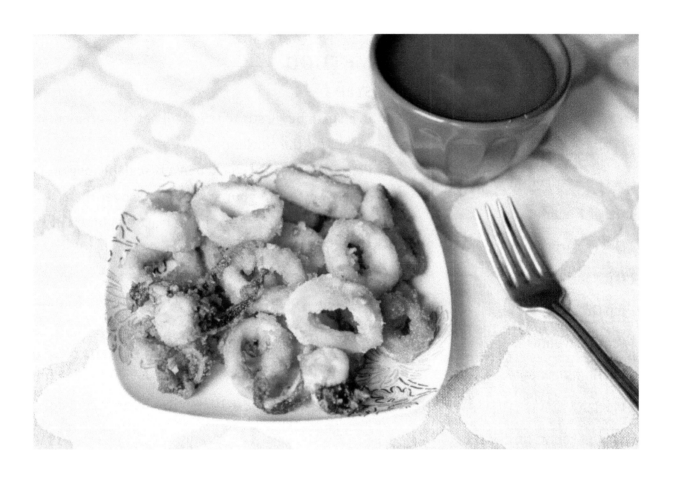

PERI CHICKEN KABOBS

Peri peri is an African spice that is popularly used for seasoning meat – in this case chicken. It is hot but not overpowering. It brings a lot of delicious seasoning to an otherwise simple meal.

MAKES 4 SERVING/ TOTAL TIME 20 MINUTE

INGREDIENTS

1.5 lbs Boneless skinless chicken breasts (cut into 1-inch pieces)

1/4 cup Apple cider vinegar

1/4 cup Extra virgin olive oil

Juice of 1 lemon

2 cloves garlic (minced)

2 tsp Paprika

1 tsp Oregano

1/2 tsp Cayenne

1 tsp Chili powder

1 tsp Salt

1/4 tsp Ground cardamom

Pinch of ginger

Freshly ground pepper (to taste)

Lime wedges (for serving)

METHOD

STEP 1

In a small bowl, stir together all of the ingredients except for the chicken.

Place the pieces of chicken in a resealable bag or shallow dish and pour the marinade over them.

Place in the refrigerator for at least two hours or overnight to marinate.

STEP 2

If using wooden skewers, soak in water for 30 minutes.

Preheat the grill to medium-high heat.

Remove the chicken from the marinade and place onto the skewers.

Grill the kebabs for 8-10 minutes or until cooked through.

Serve warm with lime wedges on the side.

NUTRITION VALUE

360 Cal, 20g fat, 4g saturated fat, 2g fiber, 39g protein, 3g carbs.

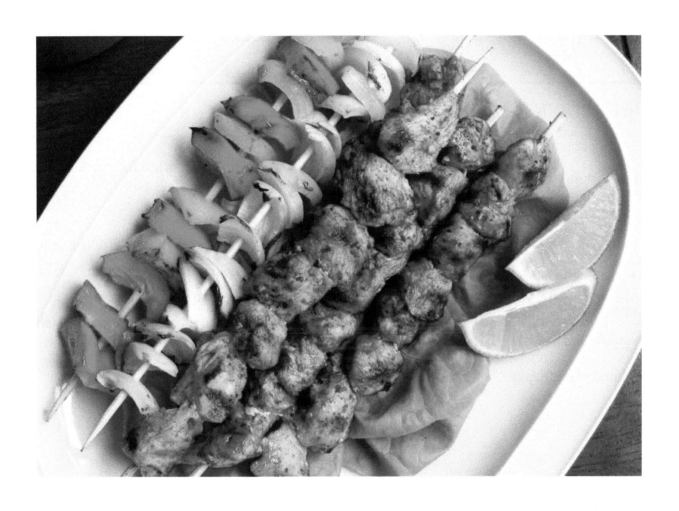

BUFFALO CHICKEN POPPERS

Great as a pretty appetizer when hosting guests, or perfect to pack for a cold lunch, these chicken poppers can easily be made when you're <u>traveling</u>.

MAKES 2 SERVING/ TOTAL TIME 20 MINUTE

INGREDIENTS

6 Mini peppers (halved)

1 c Chicken (cooked, shredded)

3 tbsp Onion (diced)

1 tbsp Louisiana Red Sauce (or your favorite "clean" hot sauce)

1 tbsp Grass fed butter (primal not paleo)

2 Hard boiled eggs (diced)

Ground black pepper (for garnish)

METHOD

STEP 1

In a small bowl, mix together shredded chicken, onion, and hardboiled eggs.

STEP 2

In a small dish, melt butter and mix it with the sauce.

Drizzle sauce over chicken mixture and combine well.

Spoon chicken mixture into pepper halves.

Garnish with fresh ground black pepper and a dash or two of red sauce.

NUTRITION VALUE

120 Cal, 5g fat, 1g saturated fat, 0.2g fiber, 21g protein, 1g carbs.

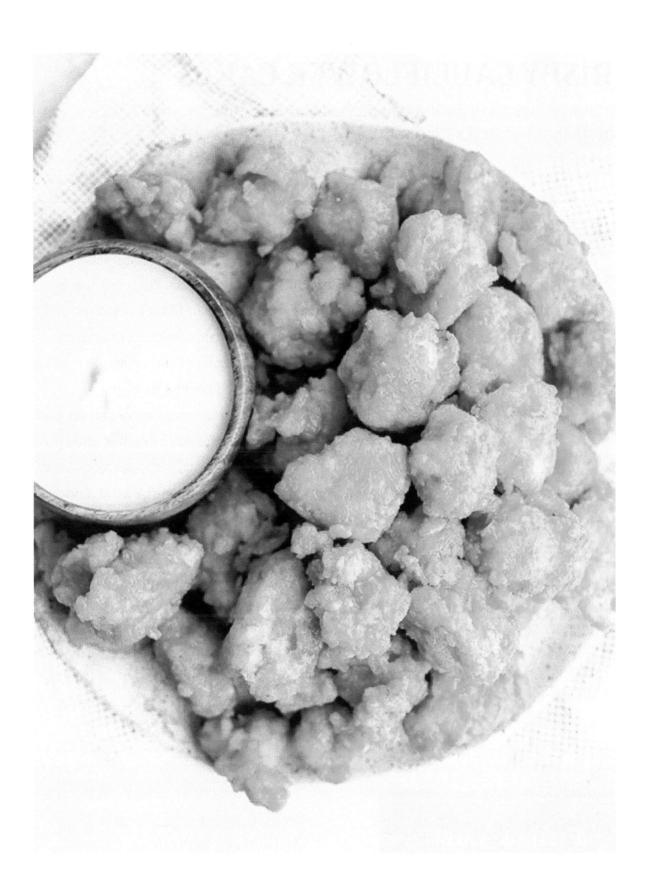

CRISPY CAULIFLOWER CAKES

Cauliflower has many health benefits such as vitamin C, vitamin K, folate, pantothenic acid, and vitamin B6.

INGREDIENTS

1 head Cauliflower

1 tbsp Ghee (or Coconut oil, melted)

2 tsp Garlic powder

2 tbsp chives (chopped)

3 tbsp Coconut flour

2 Eggs (beaten)

1 tsp Salt

2-4 tbsp Coconut oil (for frying)

METHOD
STEP 1

Cut the cauliflower into florets. Place the florets in a food processor and pulse until they become a rice like texture. Transfer the riced cauliflower to a large microwave-safe mixing bowl and microwave on high for 2 to 3 minutes, until cooked through.

Remove the bowl from the microwave and set aside to cool for about 5 minutes. Add the melted ghee (or coconut oil), chopped chives, garlic powder, coconut flour, eggs, and salt to the mixing bowl. Mix until all the ingredients are well combined.

Use your hands to form the mixture into 6 to 8 patties. Set aside.

STEP 2

Heat the coconut oil in a skillet over medium heat.

Fry the patties in the coconut oil until browned, about 2 to 3 minutes per side. Remove the patties from the oil and place on a paper towel lined plate to remove any excess oil.

NUTRITION VALUE

86 Cal, 8.7g fat, 7g saturated fat, 3g fiber, 2g protein, 6g carbs.

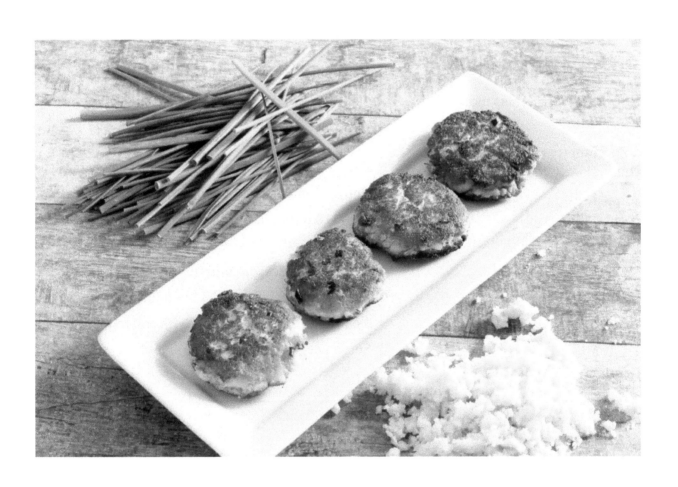

ROASTED BEETROOT HUMMUS

Roasted beets are a year-round, must-eat staple in the house. Beets are filled with good-for-you nutrients and bring out their natural sweetness when roasted.

MAKES 2 SERVING/ TOTAL TIME 45 MINUTE

INGREDIENTS

2 Beets (peeled and cut into quarters)

1/4 cup Olive oil (plus more for drizzling)

1 Zucchini (peeled and cut into chunks)

1/4 cup Tahini

1/2 Lemon (juiced)

Salt (to taste)

5-6 Carrots (peeled and cut into sticks)

METHOD

STEP 1

Preheat the oven to 400 degrees F.

Place the beet quarters on a baking sheet. Drizzle with a little olive oil and season with salt. Place in the oven and bake for 20 to 30 minutes, until the beets are fork tender. Remove from the oven and set aside to cool for about 10 minutes.

STEP 2

 In a food processor combine the roasted beets, chopped zucchini, tahini, lemon juice, and olive oil. Blend until smooth. Season with salt to taste.

 Serve with carrot sticks and enjoy!

NUTRITION VALUE

368 Cal, 19g fat, 5g saturated fat, 7g fiber, 21g protein, 14g carbs.

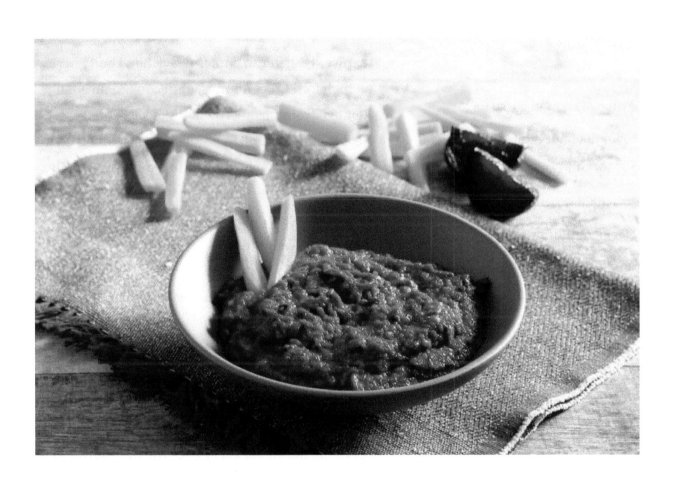

BEEF MASAMAN CURRY

There are few things more comforting than a warm bowl of delicious curry.

MAKES 3 SERVING/ TOTAL TIME 40 MINUTE

INGREDIENTS

1 1/2 lbs Skirt Steak (cut into 1 1/2 inch cubes)

1 tbsp Coconut oil

1/2 Onion (finely chopped)

3 tbsp Masaman curry paste

1 can Coconut milk

2 cups Spinach

2 tbsp Cilantro (chopped)

1 head Cauliflower

Salt (to taste)

METHOD

STEP 1

Cut the cauliflower into florets. Place the florets in a food processor and pulse until it takes on a rice like texture. Transfer to a microwave bowl and microwave on high for 3 to 4 minutes, until cooked through. Remove from the microwave and set aside.

Heat the coconut oil in a skillet over medium heat. Add the beef and brown, about 2 to 3 minutes per side. Remove from the pan and set aside.

Add the onion to the pan and sauté until translucent, about 5 to 7 minutes.

STEP 2

Add the curry paste to the pan and sauté for 1 to 2 minutes, until fragrant.

Stir in the coconut milk. Add the beef back to the pan. Add the spinach. Cover and reduce heat to a simmer. Simmer for 20 minutes. Add the fresh cilantro and season with salt to taste.

Serve the masaman curry over the cauliflower rice and enjoy!

NUTRITION VALUE

335 Kcal, 14g fat,
8g fiber, 32g protein, 14g carbs.

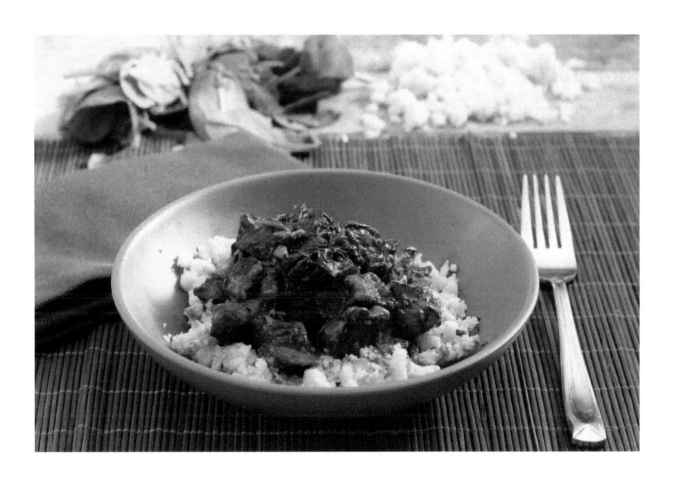

SWEET POTATO SOUP WITH BACON

Full of Thanksgiving flavors, this sweet potato soup with bacon is comfort in a bowl–plus everything is better with bacon.

MAKES 6 SERVING/ TOTAL TIME 7 HOUR

INGREDIENTS

2 lbs Sweet potatoes (peeled and roughly chopped)

2 cups Chicken stock

1 tbsp Ground cinnamon

1 tbsp Ground nutmeg

1 tsp Ground ginger

1/2 cup Coconut milk

4 slices bacon (cooked crisply and diced)

METHOD

STEP 1

Add the sweet potatoes, chicken stock, cinnamon, nutmeg, and ginger to the slow cooker.

Cook on low for 6 hours.

STEP 2

Add the coconut milk and use your immersion blender to blend until creamy.

Serve hot topped with bacon.

NUTRITION VALUE

169 Cal, 4g fat, 3g saturated fat, 5g fiber, 20g protein, 14g carbs.

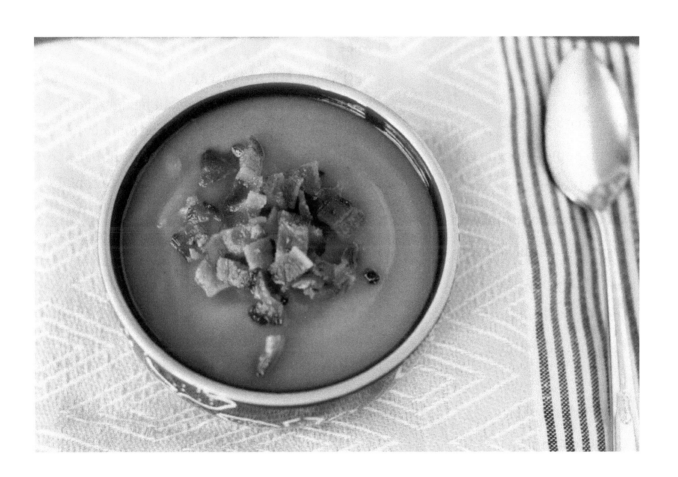

SLOW COOKER PULLED PORK

Pulled pork is one of those wonderful and delicious treats that reminds us of warm weather, picnics and hanging out with friends.

MAKES 4 SERVING/ TOTAL TIME 30 MINUTE

INGREDIENTS

2 tbsp Ghee

24 oz Tomatoes

6 oz Tomato paste

1/3 cup Apple cider vinegar

1/4 cup Honey

1/3 cup Blackstrap molasses

2 tbsp Chipotle chili powder

1 tbsp Onion powder

1 tbsp Garlic powder

2 tbsp Ground mustard

1 tsp Salt

3-4 lb Pork shoulder

1 yellow onion

1/2 cup Apple cider vinegar

1/4 cup Honey

1/3 cup olive oil

1/4 tsp Garlic powder

1/2 tsp Celery seed

METHOD

STEP 1

BBQ Sauce: Add the ghee to a pot over medium heat. Stir until melted. Add the remaining ingredients to the pot. Bring the mixture to a simmer. Simmer for 15 minutes, stirring occasionally to prevent burning. Remove from the burner and set aside to cool.

STEP 2

Pulled Pork: Pour half the BBQ sauce in the bottom of the slow cooker. Sprinkle the sliced onion on top of the sauce. Place the pork shoulder on top of the onions. Season with salt. Pour the remaining BBQ sauce over the pork. Secure the lid and cook for 8 hours on low. Once the pork is done cooking, use a fork to shred the meat.

STEP 3

Coleslaw: In a large bowl whisk together the apple cider vinegar, honey, olive oil, salt, garlic powder, and celery seed. Mix in the coleslaw vegetables.

Serve the pulled pork with the coleslaw and enjoy!

NUTRITION VALUE

415 Cal, 20g fat, 7g saturated fat, 4g fiber, 22g protein, 14g carbs.

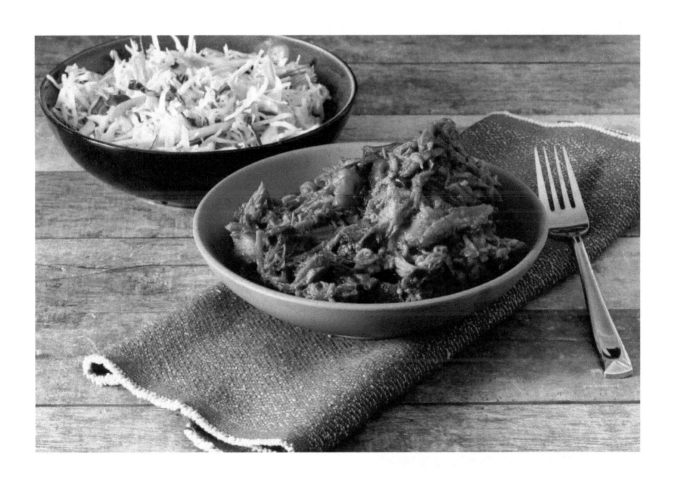

LEMON AND THYME ROASTED CHICKEN BREAST

Chicken meat is a very good source of the nutrient for the muscles – protein.

MAKES 2 SERVING/ TOTAL TIME 35 MINUTE

INGREDIENTS

2 Boneless and skinless chicken breasts

1 Lemon

6-7 Sprigs of thyme (stems discarded)

1 tbsp olive oil (plus more for drizzling)

Salt and pepper (to taste)

METHOD

STEP 1

Place the chicken in a sealable container or zip top bag. Squeeze the lemon over the chicken.

Add the thyme and olive oil. Toss to coat and season with salt. Set aside in the refrigerator for at least 30 minutes up to 8 hours.

STEP 2

Preheat the oven to 350 degrees F.

Place the chicken in a baking dish and drizzle with additional olive oil.

Bake in preheated oven for 30 minutes or until chicken is cooked.

Pepper to taste.

NUTRITION VALUE

530 Cal, 20g fat, 11g saturated fat, 7g fiber, 21g protein, 14g carbs.

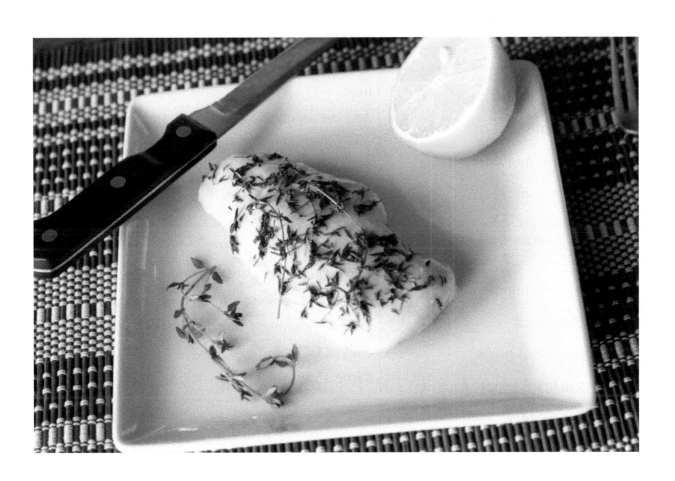

CASHEW CHICKEN

This recipe combines so many flavors that are all brought together with the cashews.

MAKES 4 SERVING/ TOTAL TIME 30 MINUTE

INGREDIENTS

2 Boneless and skinless chicken breasts (cut into 1 chunks)

1 Red bell pepper (cut into strips)

1 Onion (cut into strips)

1 Garlic cloves (minced)

1/2 cup Raw cashews

2 tbsp Coconut oil

2 tbsp Honey

1 tbsp Coconut aminos

1 tbsp Rice vinegar

1 tsp Fresh grated ginger

Sea salt and black pepper (to taste)

3 Scallions (sliced)

METHOD

STEP 1

Pour the coconut oil onto a large skillet over medium heat.

Add the onion and red pepper and cook for a few minutes.

Toss in the chicken and cook for 4 to 5 minutes.

Mix in the garlic and cashews. Cook for another 2 to 3 minutes.

STEP 2

Stir in the honey, coconut aminos, rice vinegar, grated ginger and season with salt and pepper.

Cook for another 4 to 5 minutes or until the chicken is cooked through.

Serve and garnish with scallions.

NUTRITION VALUE

91 Cal, 7g fat, 7g saturated fat, 1g fiber, 11.3g protein, 5g carbs.

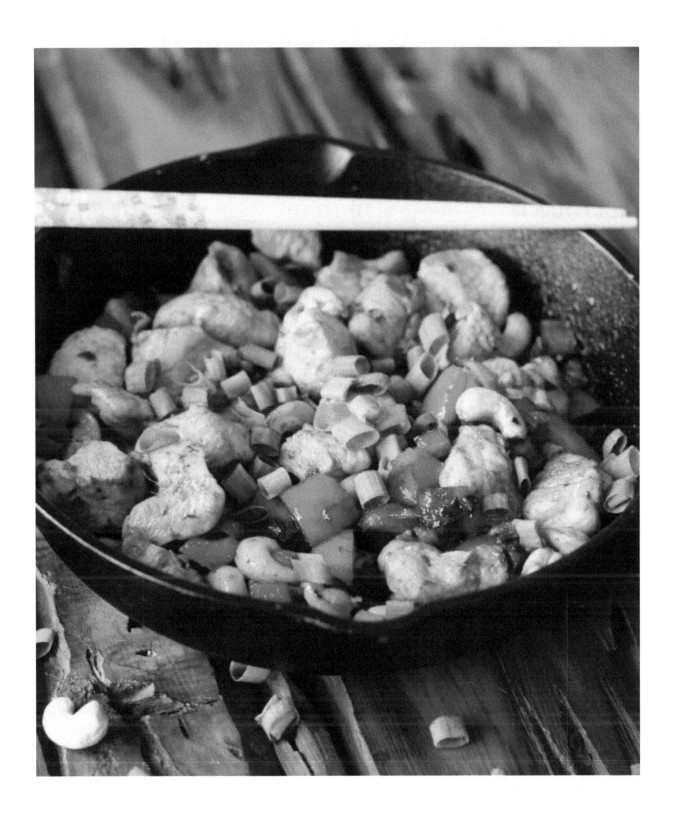

ALMOND PESTO CRUSTED COD

Cod is a good source of omega 3 and fatty acids that helps in improving the functioning of the human heart muscles, thereby keeping a person safe from the risk of an ischemic stroke.

MAKES 1 SERVING/ TOTAL TIME 15 MINUTE

INGREDIENTS

For Pesto

2 cups Arugula

3 tbsp Almonds (sliced)

1/2 Lemon (juiced)

1/4 cup olive oil

Salt (to taste)

For Fish

2 tbsp Almonds (ground)

2 tbsp Pesto

5 oz Cod

Salt (to taste)

For Noodles

1 tbsp olive oil

1 Zucchini (or 1/2 large Zucchini, spiralized or julienned)

1/4 cup Pesto

Salt (to taste)

1/4 cup Cherry tomatoes (halved

METHOD

Preheat oven to 350 degrees F.

Add the 2 tbsp of almonds to a good processor and grind. Set aside. Add the ingredients for the pesto to a food processor. Blend on high until smooth. Set aside. In a small bowl mix together the 2 tbsp almond meal and 2 tbsp of the pesto. Pat the piece of cod dry with a paper towel. Place the fish on a baking sheet. Season the fish with salt. Take the pesto and ground almonds and spoon it on top of the fish, pressing it down slightly to form a crust.

Place the fish in the oven and bake for 8-10 minutes. While the fish is cooking heat the olive oil over medium heat in a skillet. Add the zucchini noodles and ¼ cup pesto (or the rest of the pesto if it is almost gone). Sauté until the noodles are tender, about 3-4 minutes. Season with salt to taste.

Spoon the noodles onto a plate.

When the fish is done remove from the oven. Place the fish over the noodles, garnish with cherry tomatoes and serve.

NUTRITION VALUE	900 Cal, 20g fat, 20g fiber, 50g protein, 14g carbs.

42

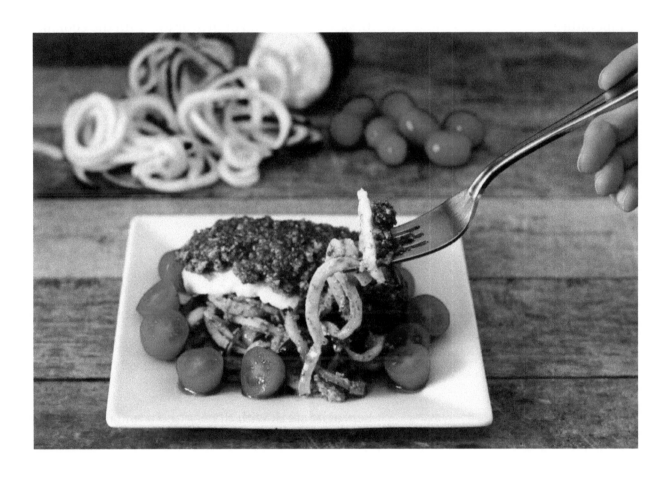

CLASSIC STEAK AND EGGS

Steak and eggs diet is really mainstream. It is probably a fact that nobody doesn't love steak and eggs.

MAKES 4 SERVING/ TOTAL TIME 25 MINUTE

INGREDIENTS

4 Steaks sirloin or T-bone, room temperature

3 tsp Cracked peppercorns fresh

1 tsp Sea salt

1 tsp Garlic powder

1 tsp Red pepper flakes

Cooking oil such as olive or coconut

6 Eggs

4 slices Tomato

METHOD

STEP 1

Grease the grill pan or grill grates with the cooking oil using a heat proof basting brush.

Heat the grill pan or outdoor grill to medium heat.

Add the peppercorn, salt, garlic powder, and pepper flakes in a bowl and combine.

Rub the spice mixture on the steak on all sides.

Add the steaks and grill for 5-7 minutes (for medium rare) or until the steak is cooked to the desired temperature.

STEP 2

Set aside to rest.

Heat coconut oil in a nonstick skillet over medium high heat.

Crack one egg at a time and cook until desired doneness.

Serve the steak with the egg and a tomato slice. Season with salt and pepper.

NUTRITION VALUE	346 Cal, 13g fat, 3g saturated fat, 2g fiber, 47g protein, 9g carbs.

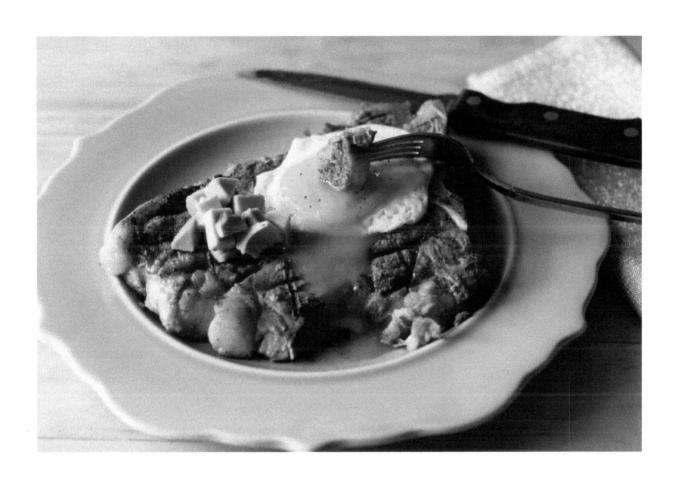

SLOW COOKER CARNE ASADA

This is the perfect Mexican inspired paleo dinner.

MAKES 4 SERVING/ TOTAL TIME 30 MINUTE

INGREDIENTS

2 lbs Sirloin steaks boneless

2 Onions diced

3 Garlic cloves minced

1 Jalapeno seeded and diced

1 Red bell pepper diced

3 Tomatoes roughly chopped

1 4 oz Green chiles diced

1/3 cup Beef broth

2 tbsp Chili powder

1 tbsp Cumin

1/4 tsp Cayenne

1/4 tsp Red pepper flake

Sea salt and black pepper to taste

8-10 Romaine leaves

METHOD

STEP 1

Season the steak with salt and pepper.

Add ½ the onion to the bottom of the slow cooker.

Place the steak on top of the onion.

Add the remaining onion, red bell pepper, jalapeno, tomato, green chiles, chili powder, cumin, cayenne, and red pepper flake.

Gently stir to combine.

STEP 2

Add the beef broth.

Set the slow cooker for 6-7 hour on low.

About 30-45 minutes before the slow cooker is done.

Remove the steak, shred with two forks and return to the slow cooker for remainder of cook time.

Serve in a romaine lettuce leaf with a side or topping of guacamole.

Other optional toppings are, homemade salsa, shredded cabbage, fresh cilantro, fresh tomatoes, paleo friendly hot sauce, and lime wedges.

NUTRITION VALUE

470 Kcal, 20g fat,
3g fiber, 21g protein, 14g carbs.

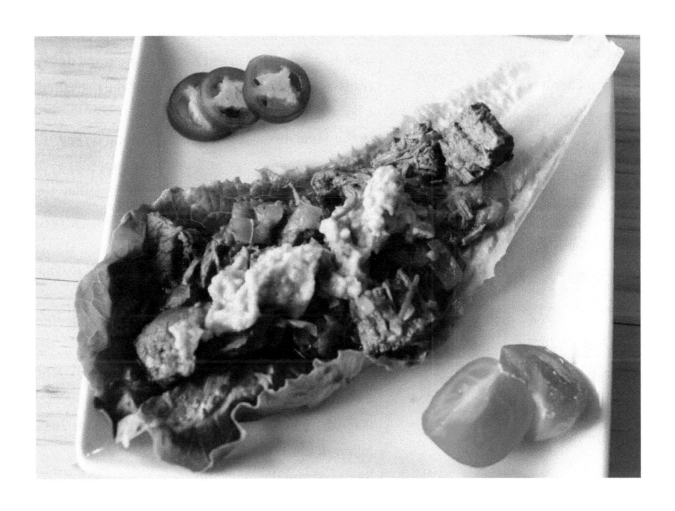

MINI PALEO MEATLOAVES

These mini paleo meatloaves are sure to be a hit at your family dinner table.

MAKES 3 SERVING/ TOTAL TIME 45 MINUTE

INGREDIENTS

1 lb Turkey

1 tbsp olive oil

1/4 Onion minced

1/4 cup Carrots diced fine

1/4 cup Green pepper diced fine

1/4 tsp Marjoram

1/4 tsp Thyme

1 Egg

1/4 tsp Salt

1/4 tsp Black pepper

1/4 cup Paleo Ketchup

6 oz Tomato paste

1/4 cup Honey

1/2 cup White wine vinegar

1/4 cup Water

3/4 tsp Salt

1/8 tsp Onion powder

1/8 tsp Garlic powder

METHOD

STEP 1

Preheat oven to 350 degrees F.

Heat the olive oil in a skillet over medium heat. Add the onions, carrots and green peppers and sauté until translucent, about 3-5 minutes. Pour the ingredients in a large mixing bowl.

In the same mixing bowl add the ground turkey, marjoram, thyme, egg, and salt and pepper.

Use your hands to mix the ingredients together, until well combined.

STEP 2

Form the meat mixture into 8-10 individual loaves and place them on a foil lined baking sheet.

In another bowl whisk together the ingredients for the paleo ketchup.

Spread some of the paleo ketchup on top of each of the individual meatloaves.

Place the meatloaves in the oven and bake for 20-25 minutes, until cooked all the way through.

Remove from the oven and serve warm

NUTRITION VALUE

255 Cal, 17g fat, 2g saturated fat, 6g fiber, 20g protein, 14g carbs.

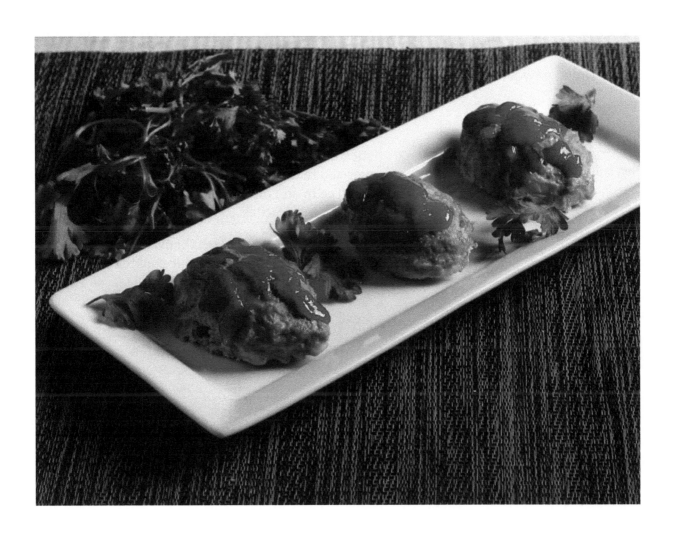

PALEO VENISON BURGERS

Burger will always be everybody's favorite. Aside from the fact that they are delicious and tasty, burgers are undeniably satisfying.

MAKES 1 SERVING/ TOTAL TIME 10 MINUTE

INGREDIENTS

1 lb Ground venison meat

1 tbsp Onion powder

1 tbsp Garlic powder

1/2 c Parsley (fresh chopped)

Sea salt and pepper (to taste)

1 c Sliced onions

1 tbsp Balsamic vinegar

1 tbsp Bacon fat (or other cooking fat)

1 Egg (optional)

METHOD

In a large mixing bowl, combine ground venison with garlic powder, onion powder, salt, pepper, and chopped parsley.

Use your hands to combine everything together and form the mixture into 4-5 patties. Please note that game meat is much less fatty than other meats, so it won't stick quite the same as other meat does. If you're worried that the patties won't stay firm while cooking, feel free to add one whisked egg to the mix before forming into patties.

Once patties are ready, set them aside and bring a large pan to high heat and melt your cooking fat. As mentioned, these suckers are quite lean, so don't skimp on the cooking fat. Bacon grease adds a really nice flavor to these burgers, in my opinion.

Once the pan is nice and hot, add the burgers, cover them, and cook them for about 3-4 minutes on each side.

Once everything is cooked through, remove the burgers from the pan and turn off the heat. Add 1 tbsp of balsamic vinegar to the onions left in the pan and deglaze the pan and drippings with the vinegar. Combine well with the onions.

Spoon caramelized onions and "gravy" over the top of the burgers and serve hot with fresh steamed veggies like asparagus!

NUTRITION VALUE	393 Cal, 20g fat, 9g saturated fat, 12g fiber, 31g protein, 14g carbs.

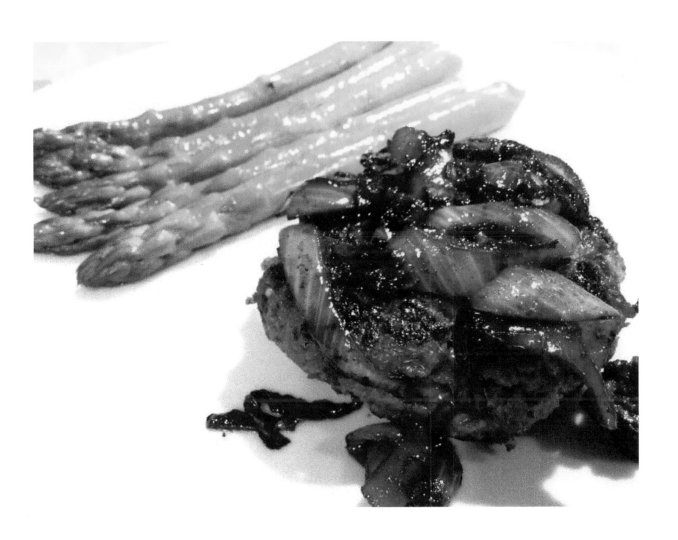

LEMON PEPPER MARINATED CHICKEN THIGHS

Weeknight chicken is no longer boring with this easy marinade!

MAKES 3 SERVING/ TOTAL TIME 30 MINUTE

INGREDIENTS

1 lb Boneless skinless chicken thighs

2 tbsp Lemon pepper seasoning (clean)

1/2 c Balsamic vinegar

1/2 c olive oil

Coconut oil

METHOD

STEP 1

In a small dish, mix together lemon pepper seasoning, vinegar, and olive oil until fully combined. Whisk until seasonings are mostly combined.

Place all chicken in a large Ziploc bag.

Add marinade to chicken in the bag and coat all the chicken pieces well by flipping and turning the bag.

Marinate in the fridge for a couple hours or overnight.

Once you're ready to cook the chicken, warm coconut oil in a medium saucepan until melted.

STEP 2

Turn up the heat, so that the pan gets nice and hot.

Lay the chicken pieces flat in the hot pan, cover, and cook for about 4-5 minutes on one side. Then flip and repeat.

Cut open a thick slice of chicken to make sure it isn't pink inside. If it's done, serve it hot with steamed veggies or cold iceberg lettuce as a side. YUM!

NUTRITION VALUE

598 Cal, 20g fat, 9g saturated fat, 13.6g fiber, 28g protein, 7g carbs.

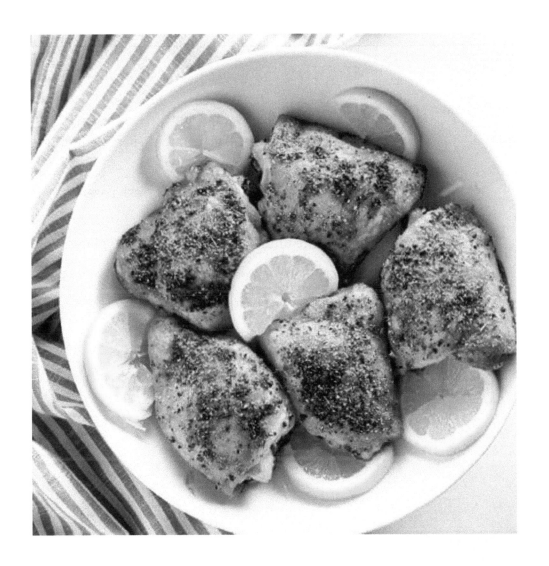

SAVORY FIG SALAD

This delicious and seasonal salad packs a paleo punch, especially when you can pick the figs right off trees in your area!

MAKES 2 SERVING/ TOTAL TIME 10 MINUTE

INGREDIENTS

1 lb Fresh figs (sliced into quarters)

1 tbsp olive oil

1 tsp Fresh rosemary (chopped)

Drizzle of honey

METHOD

STEP 1

Clean and slice fresh figs. Set aside in a medium-sized mixing bowl.

Toss fresh figs with olive oil and fresh rosemary, and drizzle with honey to taste.

Refrigerate until chilled and transfer to plates.

Serve chilled alongside grilled shrimp skewers, grilled fish, or chicken.

NUTRITION VALUE	244 Cal, 8.7g fat, 1.9g saturated fat, 13.6g fiber, 22g protein, 13g carbs.

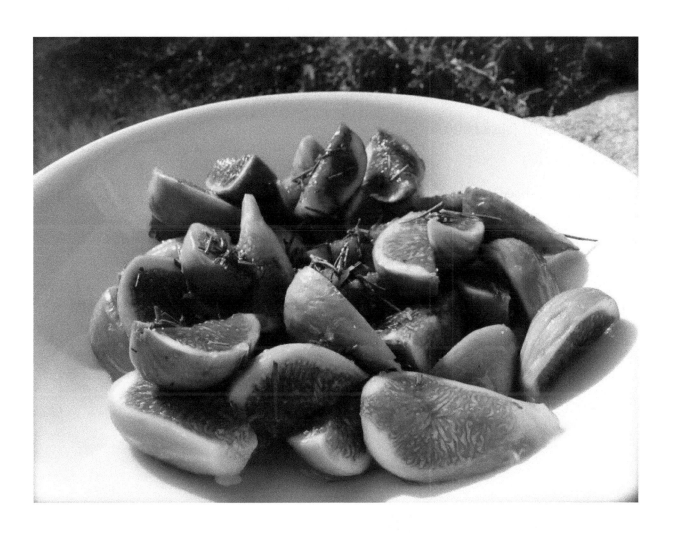

CURRY CHICKEN STIR-FRY

This super easy and healthy stir-fry gets an update with smoked paprika and red curry.

MAKES 4 SERVING/ TOTAL TIME 40 MINUTE

INGREDIENTS

2 tbsp Coconut oil

1 16 oz Broccoli florets (package frozen)

1 Red bell pepper (sliced into strips)

1 c Onion (sliced)

3 tbsp garlic (minced)

1 lb Boneless skinless chicken breasts (cut into 2 inch cubes)

1 tbsp Smoked paprika

1 tbsp Red curry powder

Cilantro (Fresh chopped - optional)

Red pepper flakes (optional)

Hot sauce (optional)

METHOD

STEP 1

In a large skillet warm coconut oil and brown chicken strips on medium until no longer pink. Set chicken aside.

In the same skillet, add onion, garlic, and broccoli. Steam on medium until tender (about 8 minutes).

Add in dry seasonings and bell pepper. Stir well to combine.

STEP 2

Add chicken chunks back in and re-heat the entire dish until bell pepper is tender but not mushy. Stir frequently.

Serve hot and add optional garnishes such as fresh chopped cilantro, red pepper flakes, or your favorite hot sauce.

NUTRITION VALUE

293 Cal, 12g fat, 8g saturated fat, 6g fiber, 31g protein, 15g carbs.

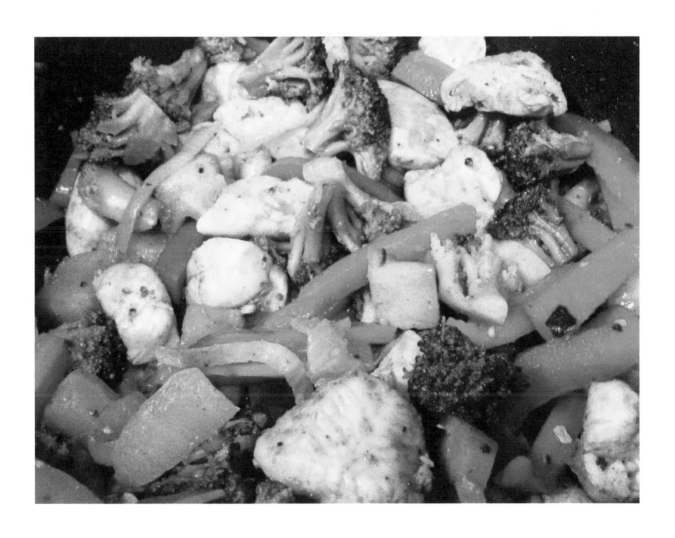

PALEO MOROCCAN CHICKEN

This would go great with some steamed Brussels sprouts or baked cabbage wedges.

MAKES 4 SERVING/ TOTAL TIME 30 MINUTE

INGREDIENTS

1 Whole chicken (cut into sections)

2-3 tbsp Bacon fat (or other cooking fat)

28 oz Tomato sauce

3 tbsp garlic (minced)

1 1/2 c Onion (diced)

1/4 Raisins (plus extra for garnish)

1/4 Alivered almonds (plus extra for garnish)

1/4 tsp Ground cinnamon

1/2 tsp Cumin

1/2 tsp Coriander

Sea salt and fresh cracked pepper (to taste)

Optional red chili flakes for garnish

Optional fresh chopped parsley for garnish

METHOD

STEP 1

Melt cooking fat on high in a large Dutch oven. Once the oil is nice and hot, sear the chicken pieces on each side for about 3 minutes and then set aside.

Reduce the heat to medium and add in onions, garlic, and a little bit of salt. Sauté until slightly caramelized, stirring frequently to prevent burning.

STEP 2

Add in tomato sauce, almonds, raisins, cinnamon, cumin, and coriander. Simmer for about 10 minutes or until flavors are fully combined.

Return the chicken to the pot and be sure that it is fully covered with sauce. Simmer on low for 45 minutes. Serve hot with sauce on top of chicken pieces and garnish with raisins, almonds, chili pepper flakes, and fresh chopped parsley.

NUTRITION VALUE

191 Cal, 8.7g fat, 1.9g saturated fat, 4g fiber, 20g protein, 14g carbs.

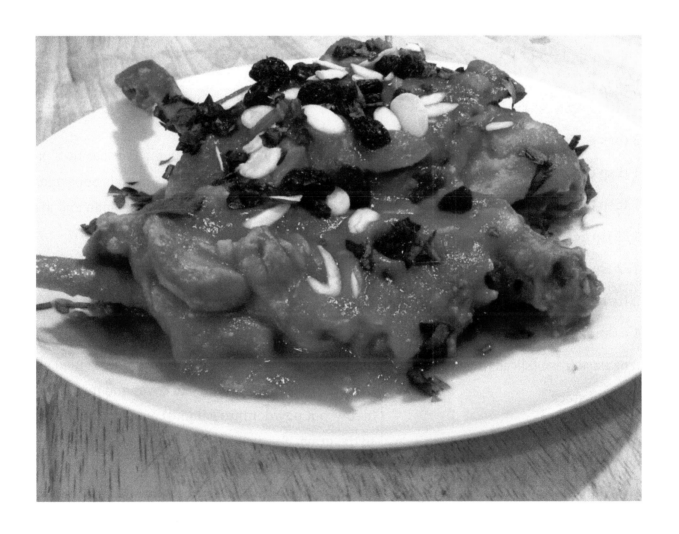

HAMBURGER STEAKS WITH STROGANOFF GRAVY

There are two secrets to making this Hamburger Steaks with Stroganoff Gravy recipe incredible: apple cider vinegar and arrowroot powder.

MAKES 4 SERVING/ TOTAL TIME 30 MINUTE

INGREDIENTS

1 lb Ground beef

3 tbsp Parsley (fresh chopped, plus extra for garnish)

3 tbsp garlic (minced)

1 tbsp Onion powder

1 tbsp Garlic powder

1/2 tsp Sea salt

1/2 tsp Fresh cracked pepper

2 tbsp Apple cider vinegar

1 c Onion (diced)

8 oz Pack fresh (sliced mushrooms)

1 c Beef stock

1 can Coconut milk

2 tbsp Arrow root powder

2 tbsp Bacon fat (or other cooking fat)

2 tbsp Grass fed butter

METHOD

STEP 1

In a large mixing bowl, mix together ground beef, parsley, minced garlic, and dry seasonings. Form into 4 patties.

In a large saucepan, melt bacon fat and sear beef patties on each side for about 2 minutes on high. Set aside.

Reduce the heat to medium in the saucepan and melt the butter. Add in onions and mushrooms. Stir frequently to prevent burning and cook until tender (about 5-8 minutes).

STEP 2

Add in beef stock, coconut milk, and apple cider vinegar. Mix 2 tbsp arrowroot powder in a small glass of water (just enough water to cover and mix the arrowroot powder into a liquid) and add the arrowroot to the gravy. Stir well.

Reduce heat and simmer on low for 20 minutes.

Add hamburger patties back to the gravy and simmer on low for another 20 minutes.

NUTRITION VALUE

471 Cal, 20g fat, 11g saturated fat, 2g fiber, 32g protein, 14.9g carbs.

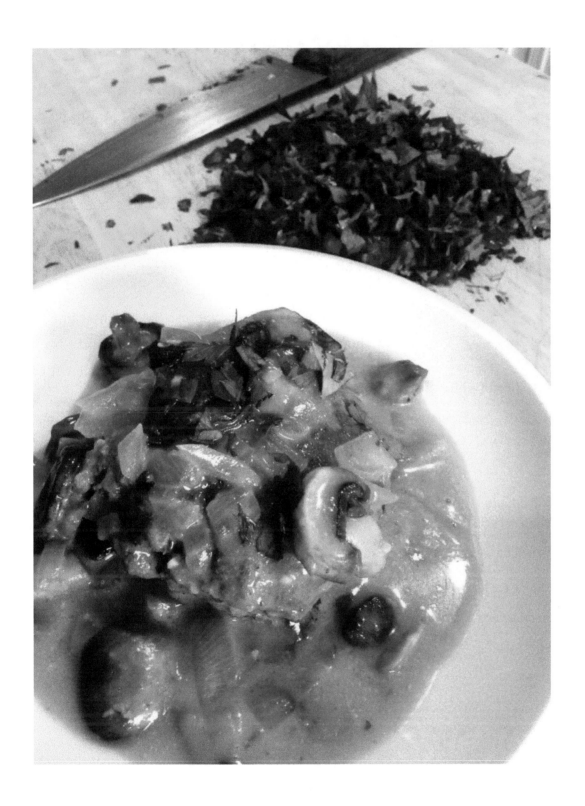

CREAM OF CAULIFLOWER & CHICKEN SOUP

This delicious and hearty soup reminds me of the creamy wild rice chicken soup .

MAKES 6 SERVING/ TOTAL TIME 20 MINUTE

INGREDIENTS

1 bag Cauliflower (frozen, about 3-4 c)

3 tbsp Coconut oil (melted)

Sea salt (to taste)

4 c Leeks (thinly sliced (white portion only))

3 tbsp garlic (minced)

3 c Mushrooms

1 tsp Thyme (dried, plus more for garnish)

3 1/4 c Bone broth*

2 c Coconut milk

2 c Cooked (shredded chicken)

Pepper (to taste)

METHOD

STEP 1

Preheat oven to 400.

Lay cauliflower florets flat on a baking sheet lined with aluminum foil or parchment paper. Drizzle 1 tbsp coconut oil over the cauliflower and sprinkle with sea salt.

Roast for 20-25 minutes, turning halfway through.

While the cauliflower is roasting, melt 2 tbsp coconut oil in a large soup pot.

STEP 2

Add in garlic and sliced leeks. Sauté until translucent. If the leeks begin to burn, feel free to add 1/4 c of water.

Once the leeks are almost done, add in thyme. Mix well.

Add bone broth, roasted cauliflower, and coconut milk. Bring to a light simmer.

Using either a regular blender or an immersion blender, blend several cups of the soup until it's smooth or until it reaches your desired consistency. I like mine hearty so I don't blend it all.

Now you can add the mushrooms and heat the soup through. Add salt and pepper to taste.

NUTRITION VALUE

335 Cal, 20g fat, 9g saturated fat, 4g fiber, 21g protein, 14g carbs.

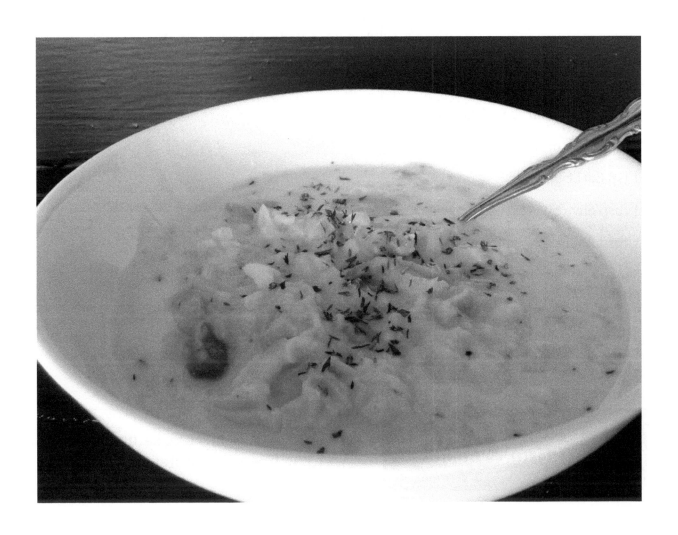

SUPER SPINACH SALAD

This easy-to-make spinach salad is bursting with flavors and antioxidants.

MAKES 4 SERVING/ TOTAL TIME 10 MINUTE

INGREDIENTS

3 c Spinach (chopped)

2 c Purple cabbage (shredded)

1 c Cucumber (sliced)

1/2 White onion (sliced_

1 c Button mushrooms (sliced)

1 tsp Onion powder

1 tsp Garlic powder

1 tbsp olive oil

1 tbsp Apple cider vinegar

Sea salt and fresh cracked pepper (to taste)

METHOD
STEP 1

Chop spinach, cabbage, cucumber, onion, and mushrooms. Toss into a large salad bowl.

Sprinkle salad with onion powder and garlic powder, salt and pepper, vinegar and oil. Toss thoroughly and gently.

NUTRITION VALUE

418 Cal, 8.7g fat, 1.9g saturated fat, 13.6g fiber, 20g protein, 14g carbs.

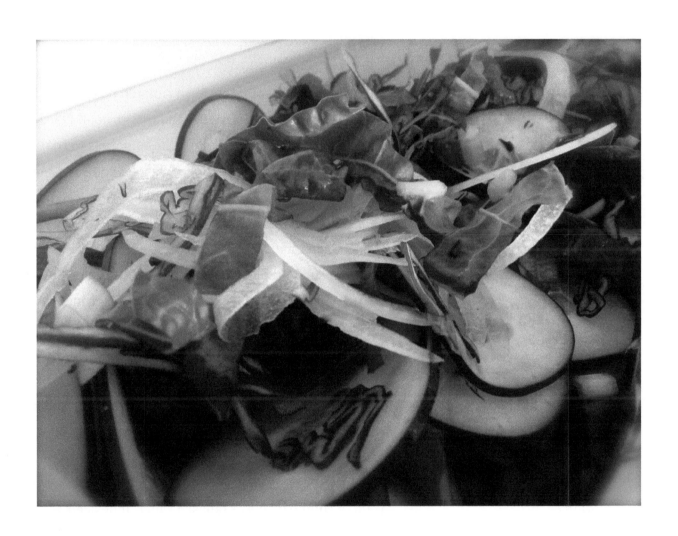

GARDEN VEGETABLE SOUP

This soup is perfect for the chilly early spring weather or for those days where you are just feeling under the weather.

MAKES 2 SERVING/ TOTAL TIME 55 MINUTE

INGREDIENTS

1 pint Grape tomatoes

3-4 tbsp Extra virgin olive oil

1/2 - 1 Onion (medium, chopped)

2 cloves garlic (minced)

1/2 bunch Asparagus (sliced at an angle into 1-inch pieces)

1 Carrot (large, peeled and sliced)

1/2 - 1 Leek (small, white part only, sliced)

4 c. Chicken broth (low-sodium)

2 tbsp Fresh chives (chopped)

1 tsp Sea salt (or as needed to season)

1 tsp Fresh ground black pepper (or as needed to season)

1/8 tsp Paleo-friendly tabasco sauce (optional)

METHOD

STEP 1

Preheat oven to 400°F.

Place the grape tomatoes on a rimmed baking sheet, drizzle on 1-2 tbsp. olive oil, and toss to coat. Place in the preheated oven and allow the tomatoes to roast for 15 minutes. Remove from the oven, let cool, and mash. Place a large skillet over medium-high heat, add in 2 tbsp. of olive oil, and let it heat up. Add in the onion, garlic, asparagus, carrot, and leek. Season with 1 tsp. each of salt and black pepper. Sauté for 2-4 minutes or until onion is translucent and garlic is fragrant.

STEP 2

Pour in the chicken broth and let simmer for 8-10 minutes or until the soup is heated through and the carrots are fork-tender. Stir in the mashed tomatoes and cook for 2 more minutes.

To serve, ladle 1 ½ - 2 c. of the soup into each soup bowl and garnish each serving with 1 tbsp. fresh chives. Add a couple drops of tabasco sauce, if desired, for added spice.

NUTRITION VALUE

289 Cal, 20g fat, 5g saturated fat, 3g fiber, 21g protein, 13g carbs.

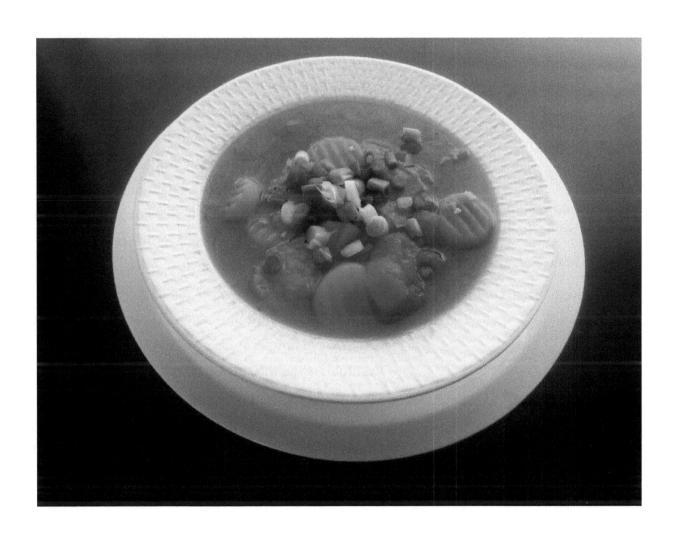

GRILLED SALMON & ZUCCHINI

This flaky salmon and sliced zucchini dish is a nutrient-packed, simple, and trouble-free dinner.

MAKES 4 SERVING/ TOTAL TIME 30 MINUTE

INGREDIENTS

2 Zucchini (large, thinly sliced (to yield 6 cups))

4 tbsp Extra virgin olive oil (divided)

2 tsp Kosher salt (divided)

1/2 tsp Fresh ground black pepper (to taste)

2 cloves garlic (minced)

1 Whole wild salmon fillet (cut into 4 equal (6 oz.) portions, 1½-lbs.)

1/3 c plus ¼ c. Fresh basil (chopped)

Your choice of paleo cooking spray

METHOD

Preheat grill to medium.

Place the sliced zucchini into a bowl with 3 tbsp. olive oil , 1 tsp. kosher salt and ½ tsp. black pepper. Toss to evenly coat the zucchini in the oil and seasonings.

Mash the minced garlic and ¾ tsp. of the salt on a cutting board) until a paste forms.

Measure out a piece of heavy-duty aluminum foil large enough for the salmon fillet. Coat the foil with cooking spray. Place the salmon skin-side down on the foil and spread the garlic mixture all over it. Sprinkle the salmon fillet with 1/3 c. basil.

Transfer the salmon on the foil to the grill. Grill for 10-12 minutes or until the salmon flakes easily and reaches an internal temperature of 145°F. Using two large spatulas, slide the salmon from the foil to a cutting board. Cut the salmon into 4 equal (6 oz.) portions.

To grill the zucchini, place the slices directly on the grill. Let grill for 5-6 minutes, then flip the slices and grill for an additional 5-6 minutes or until fork-tender.

Sprinkle each salmon fillet with a little of the remaining basil and serve.

NUTRITION VALUE	131 Cal, 15g fat, 2g saturated fat, 13.6g fiber, 21g protein, 13g carbs.

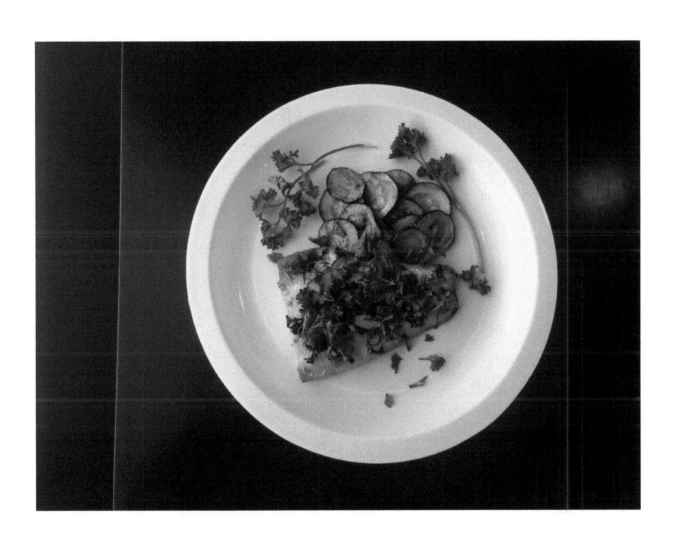

PERFECT STUFFED ZUCCHINI

Stuffed zucchini is a great option for a light yet satisfying weeknight dinner or served as a course for a dinner with friends.

MAKES 4 SERVING/ TOTAL TIME 20 MINUTE

INGREDIENTS

4 Zucchini (medium)

2 lbs Ground beef

4 Roma tomatoes (diced)

1 tbsp Extra virgin olive oil (plus more for drizzling)

1 yellow onion (medium, diced)

4 cloves garlic (minced)

1 tsp Paprika

1 tsp Ground cumin

1 tsp Salt

1/2 tsp Pepper

2 tbsp Cilantro (chopped)

METHOD

STEP 1

Preheat the oven to 375 degrees F.

Slice the zucchini in half lengthwise.

Use a spoon to scoop out the soft middle. Set aside.

Heat the tablespoon of olive oil in a large skillet over medium heat.

Add the onion and garlic to the pan and sauté for 4-5 minutes.

Add the ground beef to the pan and use a spatula to break into smaller pieces.

STEP 2

Stir in the paprika, cumin, salt, and pepper.

Cook until the beef is no longer pink, stirring occasionally.

Add the diced tomatoes to the pan and cook for 3 minutes more.

Carefully spoon the beef mixture into the zucchini.

Drizzle with olive oil and then bake for 20-25 minutes, or until the zucchini is tender.

Serve immediately, topped with chopped cilantro.

NUTRITION VALUE	664 Cal, 20g fat, 11g saturated fat, 13.6g fiber, 58g protein, 1g carbs.

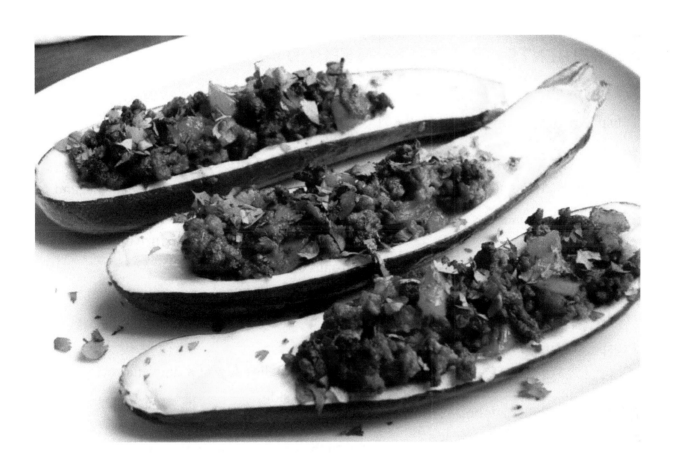

SPICY PALEO MEATBALLS IN ADOBO SAUCE

Regular meatballs are given an interesting twist with the addition of adobo sauce in this Paleo meatballs recipe.

MAKES 2 SERVING/ TOTAL TIME 20 MINUTE

INGREDIENTS

1/4 yellow onion

1 tbsp Extra virgin olive oil

1 lb Ground lamb

2 in Chipotle chilies adobo

2 cloves garlic (minced)

1/2 tsp Cumin

1/2 tsp Smoked paprika

1/2 tsp Salt

1 tbsp Coconut oil

3-4 Fresh basil leaves

2 in Chipotle chilies adobo

1 cup Tomatoes (canned diced)

1 tbsp Adobo sauce

1/2 tsp Cumin

1/2 tsp Smoked paprika

METHOD

STEP 1

Heat the olive oil in a skillet over medium heat.

Add the diced onion and sauté for 4-5 minutes until soft. Transfer to a large bowl.

Add the lamb, chilies, garlic, cumin, paprika, and salt. Stir well to fully combine.

Using your hands, form the mixture into small meatballs and set on a plate.

Melt the coconut oil in the same skillet over medium heat.

STEP 2

Add the meatballs a few at a time and cook for 3-4 minutes per side.

Once all of the meatballs have been browned, add them all into the pan and pour in the ingredients for the sauce.

Cook the meatballs in the sauce for 8-10 minutes, stirring regularly.

Serve warm and garnished with basil.

NUTRITION VALUE

803 Cal, 20g fat, 11g saturated fat, 2g fiber, 39g protein, 6g carbs.

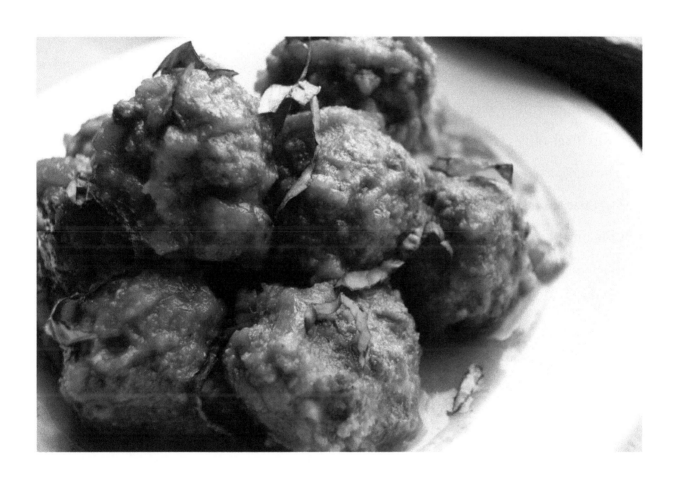

SIMPLE TACO SALAD

This taco salad can make for a healthy and substantial meal, depending on what you choose to add into it.

MAKES 2 SERVING/ TOTAL TIME 10 MINUTE

INGREDIENTS

1 Head of Romaine lettuce (chopped)

2 Roma tomatoes (thinly sliced)

1/4 Red onion (thinly sliced)

1/4 cup Black olives (sliced)

1 Avocado (pitted and diced)

1 tbsp Cilantro (chopped)

For the meat

1 lb Ground beef

2 tsp Chili powder

1 tsp Cumin

1/2 tsp Paprika

1/2 tsp Garlic powder

1/4 tsp Onion powder

1/4 tsp Oregano (dried)

Salt and freshly ground pepper (to taste)

METHOD

STEP 1

Place the lettuce, tomatoes, onion, and olives into a large bowl and toss to combine. Set aside.

Brown the ground beef in a large skillet over medium heat.

STEP 2

Stir in all of the spices.

Cook until the beef is no longer pink, stirring regularly.

To assemble, divide the lettuce mixture among the plates and top with ground beef.

Sprinkle with avocado and cilantro to serve.

NUTRITION VALUE

694 Cal, 20g fat, 17g saturated fat, 4g fiber, 59g protein, 8g carbs.

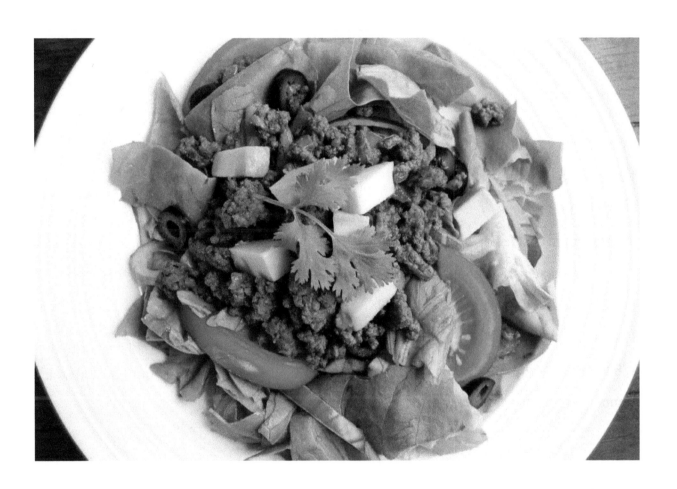

LEMON AND ROSEMARY GRILLED CHICKEN

This recipe is a simple but tasty way to prepare chicken using ingredients that you probably already have on hand.

MAKES 3 SERVING/ TOTAL TIME 40 MINUTE

INGREDIENTS

1 lb Boneless and skinless chicken breasts

3 tbsp Extra virgin olive oil

4 cloves garlic (minced)

1 tbsp Lemon juice

1 tbsp Lemon zest

2 tsp Fresh rosemary (chopped)

1/4 tsp Red pepper flakes

1/4 tsp Salt

1/8 tsp Freshly ground pepper

Lemon wedges (for garnish)

METHOD

STEP 1

To make the marinade, stir together the olive oil, garlic, lemon juice and zest, rosemary, red pepper flakes, salt, and pepper in a small bowl.

Place the chicken in a resealable bag or shallow dish and pour the marinade over it.

STEP 2

Place in the refrigerator for at least three hours (overnight, if you wish) to marinate.

Preheat the grill to medium-high.

Drain the marinade and place the chicken onto the grill.

Cook for 7-8 minutes per side or until the chicken is no longer pink.

Garnish with lemon wedges to serve.

NUTRITION VALUE

313 KJ Energy, 17g fat, 2g saturated fat, 2g fiber, 36g protein, 4g carbs.

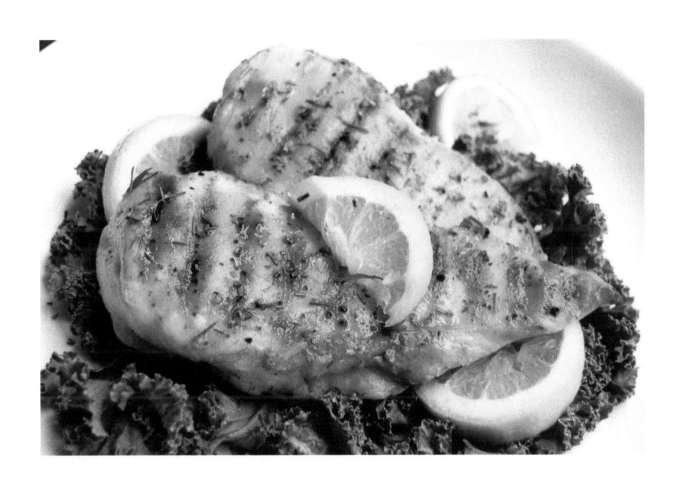

COCONUT CHICKEN STRIPS WITH A HONEY MUSTARD DIPPING SAUCE

This recipe is perfect for little fingers that want to help out in the kitchen!

MAKES 2 SERVING/ TOTAL TIME 30 MINUTE

INGREDIENTS

2 Chicken breasts (sliced into strips)

1/2 c Coconut flour

2 Eggs

1 c Unsweetened coconut flakes

Vegetables (optional)

Honey Mustard Dipping Sauce

1/2 c Honey

1/2 c Dijon mustard

METHOD

STEP 1

Line a baking sheet with parchment paper and preheat the oven to 400 degrees F.

Wash the chicken breasts and slice them into strips. Pat them dry with a paper towel and set them aside.

Put the coconut flour onto a medium-sized plate. Set it aside. Whisk the 2 eggs in a medium-sized bowl. Set it aside. Put the coconut flakes onto a medium-sized plate and set it aside.

STEP 2

Carefully dip the chicken strips first into the flour, then into the eggs, and finally into the coconut flakes. Place the strips gently onto the baking sheet lined with parchment paper.

Bake for about 15 minutes or until the strips are brown. While baking, mix up a batch of Honey Mustard Dipping Sauce using equal parts honey and Dijon mustard.

Once complete, drizzle the honey mustard over the chicken strips and serve with your favorite steamed veggies.

NUTRITION VALUE	369 Cal, 20g fat, 7g saturated fat, 28g fiber, 21g protein, 14g carbs.

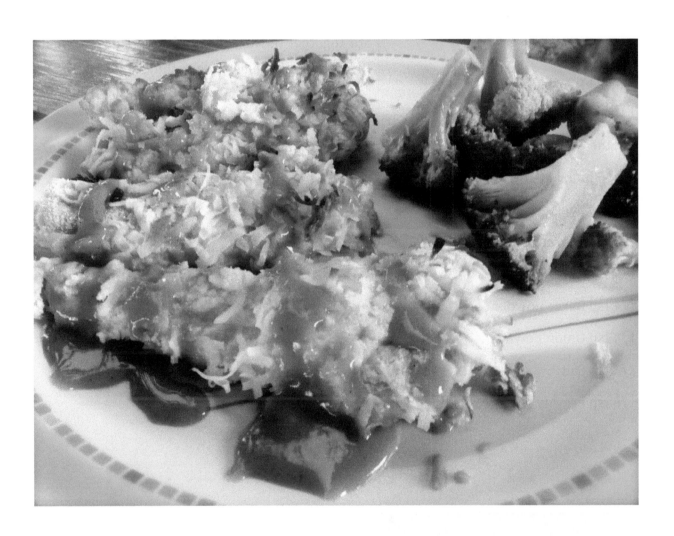

PAN-SEARED CAJUN SALMON

Pan seared Salmon is a very quick and simple weeknight meal and it's ready in less than fifteen minutes.

MAKES 2 SERVING/ TOTAL TIME 30 MINUTE

INGREDIENTS

2 6- oz Salmon fillets

1 tbsp Coconut oil

1 tbsp Cilantro (chopped)

For the Cajun rub

1 tsp Smoked paprika

1/2 tsp Oregano (dried)

1/2 tsp Thyme (dried)

1/4 tsp Cayenne

1/4 tsp Garlic powder

1/4 tsp Onion powder

1/4 tsp Salt

1/8 tsp Freshly ground pepper

METHOD

Stir together the ingredients for the rub in a small bowl.

Rub into the (skinless side of the) salmon.

Melt the coconut oil in a non-stick skillet over medium-high heat.

Place the salmon in the pan with the skin side up.

Sear for 3-4 minutes until browned.

Carefully flip over and cook for an additional 3-5 minutes or until the salmon reaches your desired level of doneness.

Serve warm and garnished with cilantro.

NUTRITION VALUE

360 Cal, 20g fat, 4g saturated fat, 2g fiber, 39g protein, 3g carbs.

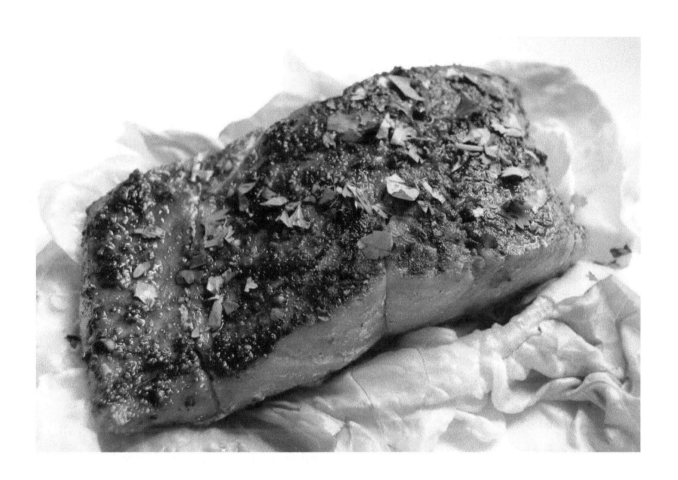

PALEO TACO SEASONING AND SALAD

Homemade Paleo Taco Seasoning just taste better that those that can be bought in stores. It is one of our favorite meal and we'll be sharing you our secret recipe!

MAKES 4 SERVING/ TOTAL TIME 10 MINUTE

INGREDIENTS

Seasoning

2 tsp Chili powder

2 tsp Cumin

1 tsp Salt

2 tsp Garlic powder

2 tsp Onion powder

Salad

1 lb Ground beef

1 Onion (small, diced)

1/4 Head iceberg lettuce (chopped)

1 Avocado (diced)

1 Tomato (diced)

METHOD

STEP 1

Combine all the seasonings in a ramekin and mix well. You might consider doubling or tripling the batch and setting the taco seasoning aside in the pantry for future use. In a large sauté pan, begin sautéing the ground beef on medium.

STEP 2

Add the seasonings to the beef and mix well while browning.

While browning, chop up other ingredients. You might consider creating a self-serve taco bar by placing each ingredient in a small serving bowl and allowing your guests to pick their own ingredients.

Once the beef is done, serve it on top of the iceberg lettuce and garnish it with your desired toppings. No dressing needed!

NUTRITION VALUE

346 Cal, 20g fat, 8g saturated fat, 1g fiber, 30g protein, 6g carbs.

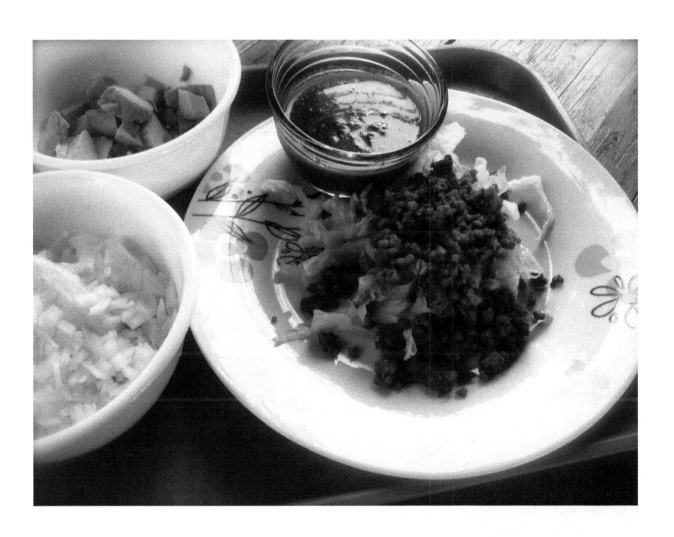

ROASTED RADISHES AND ASPARAGUS

This simple recipe makes great use of extra spring vegetables.

MAKES 2 SERVING/ TOTAL TIME 20 MINUTE

INGREDIENTS

3 cups Radishes (halved)

3 tbsp Extra virgin olive oil (divided)

2 tsp Salt (divided)

Freshly ground pepper (to taste)

3 tbsp Fresh rosemary (chopped)

1 Bunch Asparagus (chopped)

METHOD

STEP 1

Preheat the oven to 425 degrees F.

Place the radishes in a large bowl and toss with 2 tablespoons of olive oil.

Add half of the salt and rosemary and sprinkle with pepper.

Toss well to coat.

STEP 2

Place onto a rimmed baking sheet and bake for 15 minutes.

Meanwhile, toss the asparagus with the remaining tablespoon of olive oil and rosemary.

After the radishes have been baking for 15 minutes, add the asparagus to the baking sheet and bake everything for 15-20 minutes more, until the radishes are browned and crisp.

Serve immediately.

NUTRITION VALUE	350 Cal, 26g fat, 5g saturated fat, 17g fiber, 21g protein, 26g carbs.

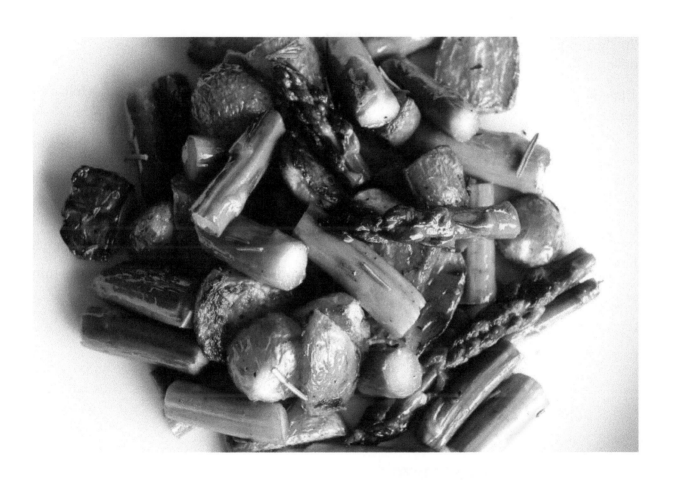

GARLIC JALAPEÑO SHRIMP

It's very easy to get bored with eating paleo if you stick to eating the more common meats like chicken and beef.

MAKES 2 SERVING/ TOTAL TIME 40 MINUTE

INGREDIENTS

20 Shrimp (medium-sized, peeled and deveined)

1 Jalapeno (diced, with ribs and seeds removed)

1 tbsp Coconut oil

1 tbsp garlic (minced)

Sea salt and fresh cracked pepper (to taste)

Fresh lemons (optional)

METHOD

STEP 1

Peel, devein, and clean shrimp. Set aside.

Warm coconut oil in a medium saucepan while dicing jalapeño.

Add minced garlic to the warm coconut oil in the pan.

Allow it to become fragrant (about 3 minutes on medium).

STEP 2

Add shrimp and jalapeño to the pan. Cook shrimp for about 3-5 minutes or until shrimp is white and fully cooked.

Serve with fresh lemons.

Enjoy!

NUTRITION VALUE	822 Cal, 19g fat, 1.9g saturated fat, 10g fiber, 20g protein, 13g carbs.

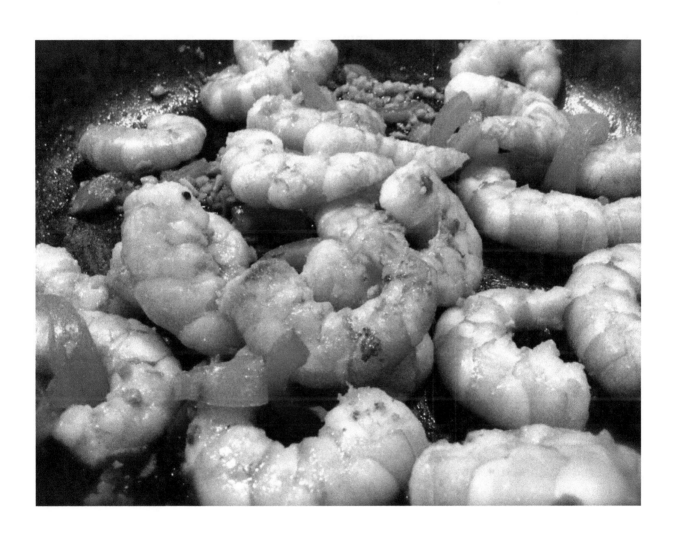

SPICY FISH CURRY SOUP

Summer is the season of fish! Use this recipe for whatever fresh or salt-water haul you bring home. It's great as a starter or as a main dish.

MAKES 2 SERVING/ TOTAL TIME 20 MINUTE

INGREDIENTS

1 lb White fish fillet (cleaned and cut into 1 inch cubes)

2 c Bone broth*

4 tbsp Red curry paste

1 can Coconut milk

2 Carrots (diced)

1 c Red cabbage (sliced)

2 Zucchinis (small, diced)

1/2 c Onion (diced)

3 tbsp garlic (minced)

1 tbsp Coconut oil

1 tsp Salt

1 c Fresh cilantro (chopped (as garnish))

Powdered cayenne (to taste (optional))

Paleo-friendly sriracha** (optional)

METHOD

STEP 1

In a large soup pot, sauté diced onions and garlic in coconut oil on medium until translucent and fragrant. Add in bone both and red curry paste. Mix well.

Once bone broth and curry are well combined, stir in remaining vegetables (carrots, cabbage, and zucchini). Bring to a strong simmer and simmer for about 20 minutes.

STEP 2

Turn down heat and add coconut milk, salt, and fish. Simmer on low for another 10 minutes or until fish turns white.

Serve hot with a sprinkle of cayenne, paleo-friendly sriracha**, and/or chopped fresh cilantro.

NUTRITION VALUE

189 Cal, 6g fat, 4g saturated fat, 3g fiber, 24g protein, 11g carbs.

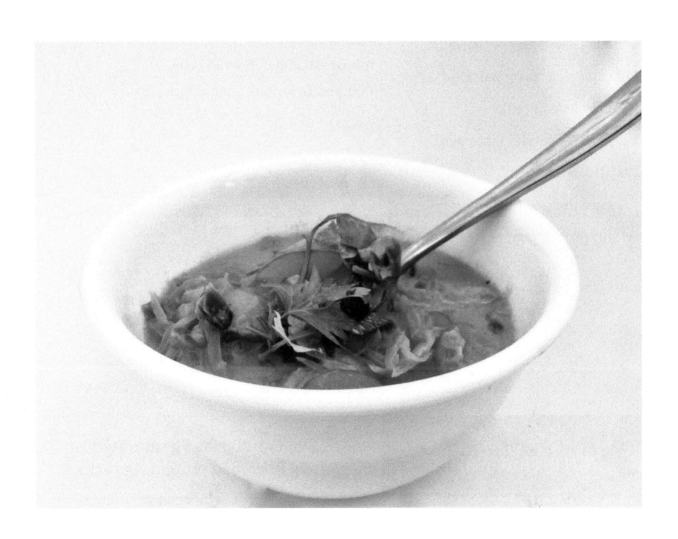

EASY CHICKEN SALAD

Chicken salad is one of the simplest paleo lunch recipes to put together.

MAKES 4 SERVING/ TOTAL TIME 10 MINUTE

INGREDIENTS

5 cups Chicken breast (cooked, shredded)

1 1/2 cups Red grapes (halved)

1/3 cup Paleo mayonnaise

1 Stalk celery (diced)

2 tbsp Fresh parsley (chopped)

2 tsp Dijon mustard

1/2 tsp Salt

Freshly ground pepper (to taste)

METHOD

STEP 1

Combine all of the ingredients in a large bowl and stir well to combine.

Adjust salt and pepper to taste.

Refrigerate for one hour before serving.

NUTRITION VALUE	596 Cal, 20g fat, 7g saturated fat, 1g fiber, 88g protein, 4g carbs.

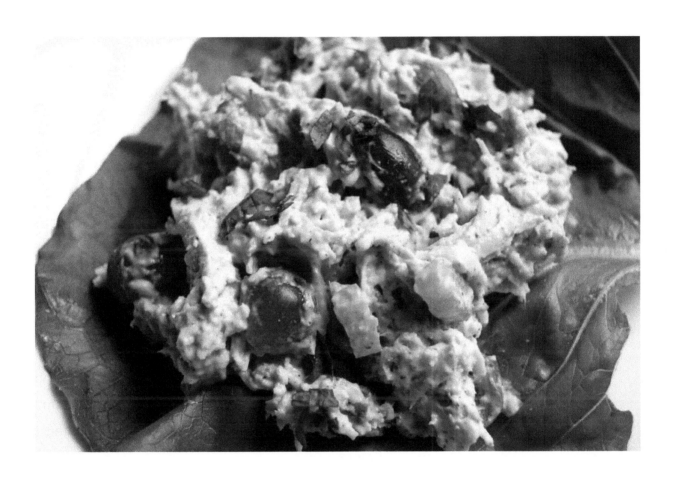

CURRIED CARROT SOUP

Coconut milk and curry bring a tasty twist to regular carrot soup in this recipe.

INGREDIENTS

2 lbs Carrots (peeled and roughly chopped)

2 tbsp Extra virgin olive oil

1/2 White onion (large , roughly chopped)

1 tsp Curry powder

3 cloves garlic (minced)

5 cups Vegetable stock

1/2 cup Coconut milk

Salt and pepper (to taste)

METHOD

STEP 1

Heat the olive oil in a large saucepan over medium heat.

Add the onion, curry powder, and a pinch of salt.

Sauté for 4-5 minutes.

Add the garlic and cook for one minute more.

Add the carrots and stock into the pot.

Bring to a boil, and then reduce the heat to simmer.

Simmer, covered, for 18-20 minutes until the carrots are tender.

STEP 2

Remove from heat.

Use an immersion blender to purée the ingredients in the pot until smooth.

Alternatively, transfer to a blender in batches to purée.

Return the puréed soup to the stove over medium heat and stir in the coconut milk, cooking for 3-4 minutes more.

Adjust salt and pepper to taste. Serve warm.

NUTRITION VALUE

215 Cal, 13g fat, 6g saturated fat, 7g fiber, 22g protein, 14g carbs.

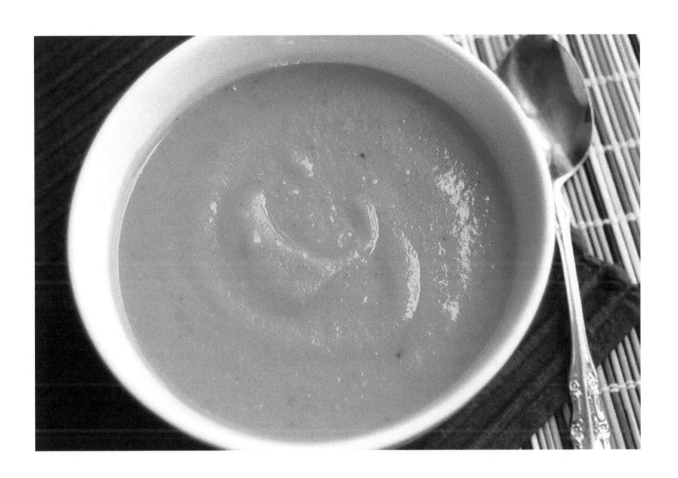

PERFECT COBB SALAD

Cobb salad comes in many varieties, but is always a hearty and satisfying meal.

MAKES 4 SERVING/ TOTAL TIME 10 MINUTE

INGREDIENTS

1 Head romaine lettuce (chopped)

6 Eggs

8 slices bacon

1/2 cup Slivered almonds

1/2 Red onion (diced)

1 cup Cherry tomatoes (chopped)

For the dressing

3/4 cup Extra virgin olive oil

1 tbsp Red wine vinegar

1 tsp Lemon juice

1/4 tsp Dry mustard

Dash of honey

1 clove garlic (minced)

Salt and freshly ground pepper (to taste)

METHOD

STEP 1

Place the eggs in a saucepan and add enough cold water to cover them by an inch.

Bring the water to a boil and then remove the pot from heat and cover.

Let stand for 10 minutes and then place the eggs into a bowl of ice water for 1-2 minutes.

Crack and peel the shells off the eggs.

Slice thinly and set aside.

STEP 2

Meanwhile, cook the bacon in a skillet until crisp.

Remove to a paper towel-lined plate and crumble.

To make the dressing, combine all of the dressing ingredients together in a blender.

Blend until smooth. Season to taste with salt and pepper.

To assemble the salad, divide the romaine lettuce among the plates. Top evenly with sliced eggs, crumbled bacon, almonds, tomatoes, and onions. Serve with dressing on the side.

NUTRITION VALUE

573 Cal, 20g fat, 7g saturated fat, 5g fiber, 21g protein, 8g carbs.

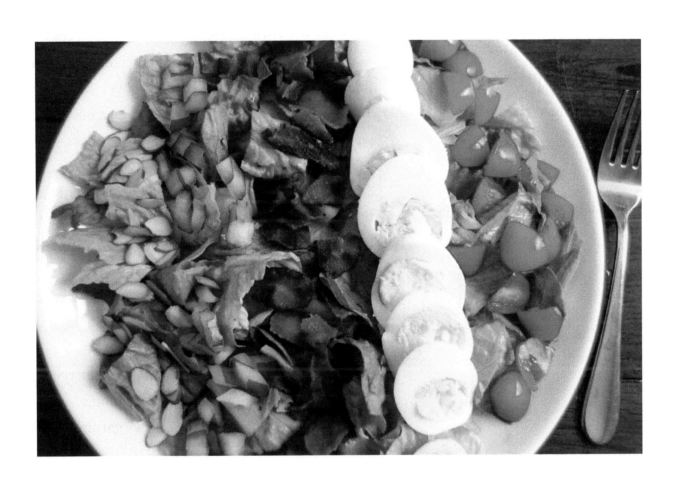

CLASSIC EGG SALAD

This recipe provides the guidelines for making the Classic Egg Salad, which is extremely paleo at heart.

MAKES 3 SERVING/ TOTAL TIME 20 MINUTE

INGREDIENTS

6 Eggs

1/4 cup Red onion (finely diced)

1 Stalk celery (finely diced)

2 Green onions (chopped)

1/4 cup Paleo mayonnaise

2 tsp Dijon mustard

Salt and freshly ground pepper (to taste)

METHOD

STEP 1

Place the eggs in a saucepan and add enough cold water to cover them by an inch. Bring the water to a boil and then remove the pot from heat and cover. Let stand for 10 minutes and then place the eggs into a bowl of ice water for 1-2 minutes.

Crack and peel the shells off the eggs.

Separate the yolks from the egg whites. Discard half of the egg yolks and place the remaining ones into a small bowl.

STEP 2

Stir together the egg yolks, mayonnaise, mustard, salt, and pepper.

Finely dice the egg whites.

Place them in a separate bowl along with the red onion, celery, and green onions and stir to combine.

Stir in the mayonnaise mixture. Serve garnished with additional green onions if desired.

NUTRITION VALUE	245 Kcal, 18g fat, 3g fiber, 20g protein, 15g carbs.

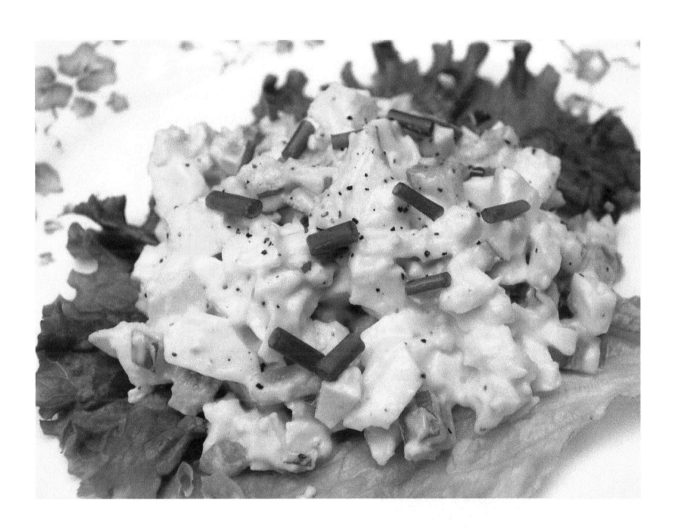

ASPARAGUS SPRING SALAD WITH DILL

This crunchy, light salad is tossed with a simple dill dressing, which adds a delicious and tangy flavor.

MAKES 4 SERVING/ TOTAL TIME 20 MINUTE

INGREDIENTS

1 lb Asparagus (trimmed and chopped)

4 Radishes (thinly sliced)

2 Stalks celery (finely diced)

1 Head romaine lettuce (chopped)

For the dressing

1 tbsp Lemon juice

1 Shallot (minced)

1 tbsp Fresh dill (chopped)

1 tsp Dijon mustard

1/8 tsp Salt

1/4 cup Extra virgin olive oil

METHOD

STEP 1

Bring a pot of salted water to a boil.

Add the asparagus and blanch for 2-3 minutes. It should be just barely cooked through and still crisp.

Prepare a large bowl of ice water while the asparagus is cooking.

STEP 2

Remove the asparagus from the hot water and place into the ice bath. Drain and pat dry with a paper towel.

To make the dressing, whisk together the lemon juice, shallot, dill, mustard, and salt. Drizzle in the olive oil, whisking continuously until smooth.

Combine the asparagus, radishes, celery, and lettuce in a large bowl. Pour the dressing over the salad and toss to evenly coat.

Serve immediately.

NUTRITION VALUE

154 Cal, 15g fat, 2g saturated fat, 3g fiber, 23g protein, 5g carbs.

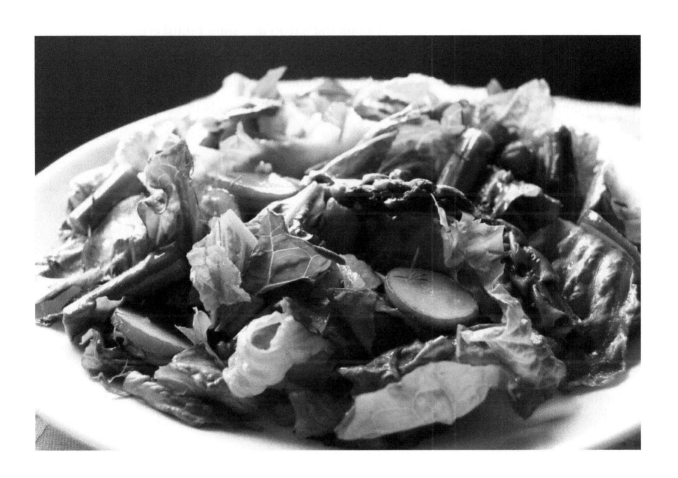

BRILLIANT BROCCOLI SALAD

This easy raw broccoli salad is the perfect side dish for summer picnics and barbecues.

MAKES 5 SERVING/ TOTAL TIME 30 MINUTE

INGREDIENTS

2 Heads of broccoli (cut into florets)

1 Red apple (large, diced)

3/4 cup Slivered almonds

1/2 cup Raisins

3 slices bacon

For the dressing

1/4 cup Extra virgin olive oil

2 tbsp Honey

1 tbsp Dijon mustard

1 tbsp White wine vinegar

2 cloves garlic (peeled)

Juice of 1 lemon

Salt and freshly ground pepper (to taste)

METHOD

STEP 1

Cook the bacon in a skillet until crisp.

Remove from the pan to a paper towel-lined plate. Crumble and set aside.

Lightly toast the almonds in a separate skillet over medium heat until golden. Set aside to cool.

STEP 2

Place all the ingredients for the dressing into a blender or food processor and purée until smooth. Adjust salt and pepper to taste.

Add the broccoli, apple, and raisins into a large bowl and stir to combine.

Add the bacon and almonds.

Drizzle in the dressing and stir well to coat.

Refrigerate for one hour before serving.

NUTRITION VALUE

398 Cal, 20g fat, 3g saturated fat, 5g fiber, 22g protein, 14g carbs.

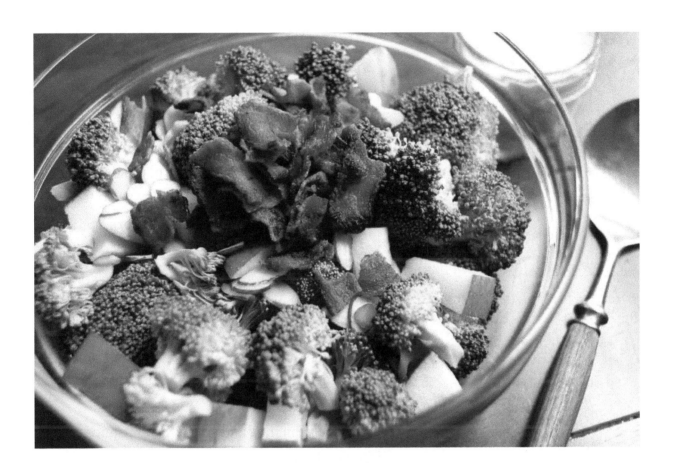

PALEO VEGETABLE CURRY

The paleo diet has plenty of vegetarian-friendly options, including this delicious, spicy curry.

INGREDIENTS

1 tbsp Coconut oil

2 tbsp Panaeng curry paste

1 yellow onion (medium, diced)

4 cloves garlic (minced)

1/2 Red bell pepper (thinly sliced)

1/2 yellow bell pepper (thinly sliced)

1 Yellow squash (small, chopped)

1 Head of broccoli (small, cut into florets)

1 14 oz can Coconut milk

1 tsp Coconut aminos

Salt (to taste)

2 tsp Lime juice

1/4 cup Cilantro (chopped)

METHOD

STEP 1

Melt the coconut oil in a large pan over medium heat.

Add the curry paste and cook for 2-3 minutes, stirring frequently.

Add the onion and garlic to the pan, along with a dash of salt, and sauté for 4-5 minutes.

Stir in the bell peppers, squash, and broccoli.

Sauté for 2-3 minutes more.

STEP 2

Add the coconut milk and coconut aminos to the pan and bring to a simmer.

Cook for 10-15 minutes until the coconut milk has thickened slightly and the vegetables are tender.

Adjust salt to taste.

Remove from heat and stir in the lime juice.

Top with cilantro to serve.

NUTRITION VALUE

331 Kcal, 20g fat, 5g fiber, 22g protein, 13g carbs.

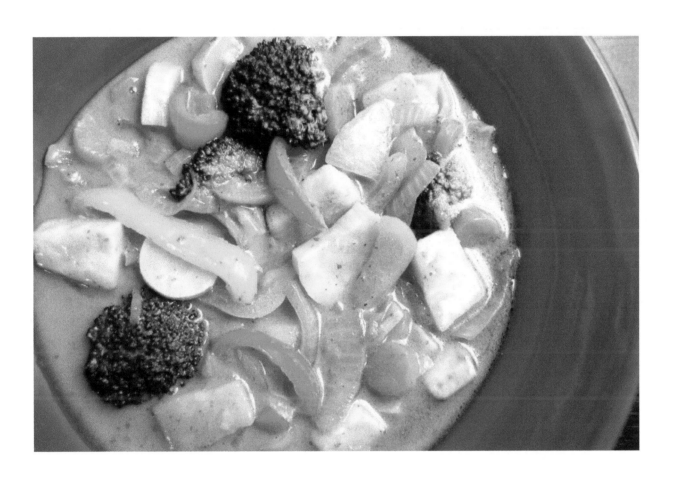

VEGETABLE SOUP WITH CABBAGE AND ONION "NOODLES"

That's a healthy bunch of ingredients. In this cuisine, you will learn how to prepare it for yourself.

MAKES 6 SERVING/ TOTAL TIME 30 MINUTE

INGREDIENTS

4 c Bone broth*

1 c White onion (very thinly sliced, use a mandolin slicer)

1 c Cabbage (very thinly sliced)

1/2 c Carrots (chopped)

1/2 c Spinach (chopped)

1 tbsp garlic (minced)

1/2 tbsp Coconut oil

Salt and pepper (to taste)

1 Bay leaf

METHOD

STEP 1

Add coconut oil and minced garlic to soup pot. Warm until fragrant.

Add bone broth to soup pot and turn up heat to bring soup to a slight simmer.

Add cabbage, onions, carrots, and bay leaf. Simmer for 20 minutes.

STEP 2

Once onions, cabbage, and carrots are fully cooked but not mushy, add in spinach. Simmer 5 minutes longer.

Taste test the soup and add salt and pepper. Remember, the bone broth has not been salted, so you might have to be generous with the salt.

Garnish with paleo-approved hot sauce.

NUTRITION VALUE	471 Cal, 20g fat, 11g saturated fat, 2g fiber, 32g protein, 14.9g carbs.

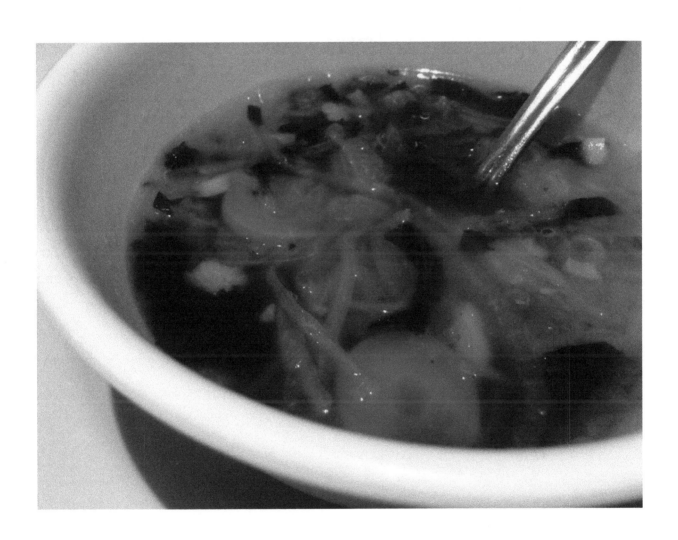

PALEO PULLED PORK & BROCCOLI

This slow cooker dish takes boring pork and turns it into an exciting dinner in just a few steps.

MAKES 4 SERVING/ TOTAL TIME 30 MINUTE

INGREDIENTS

1 lb Pork (feel free to use a cut that would be too tough to cook any other way)

1/2 c Onions (shredded)

1/2 c Cabbage (shredded)

1 tsp Garlic powder

1 tsp Onion powder

Sea salt and fresh ground pepper (to taste)

1/2 c Water

1 c Broccoli florets

Cayenne pepper (optional)

Coconut aminos (optional)

Ginger (Fresh grated - optional)

METHOD

STEP 1

Add everything but broccoli to Crock-Pot and cook on low for 8 hours or until pork falls off easily.
Once the pork is done, use 2 forks to shred the meat and mix everything together.

STEP 2

Add broccoli florets into the Crock-Pot for about 15 minutes or until they are steamed and warmed through.
Garnish with cayenne pepper, coconut aminos, and fresh grated ginger.

NUTRITION VALUE

355 Cal, 19g fat, 7g saturated fat, 3g fiber, 34g protein, 10g carbs.

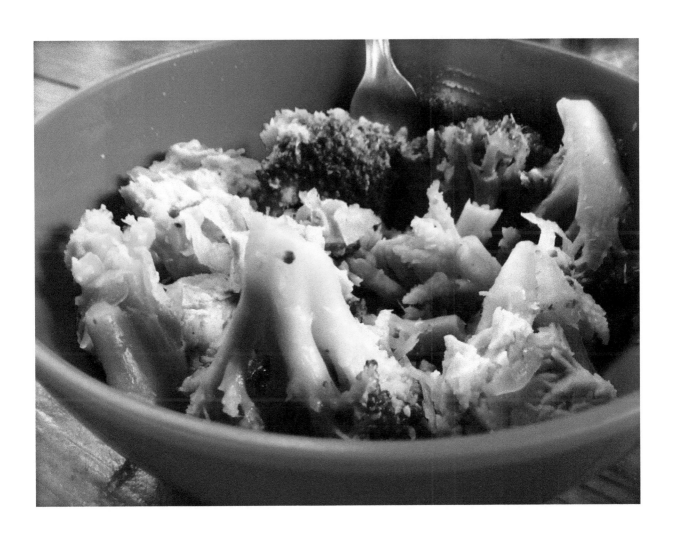

Lightning Source UK Ltd.
Milton Keynes UK
UKHW051434100621
385263UK00002B/325